BLOOD TYPE O DIET COOKBOOK

Complete Guide for Optimal Health and Wellness Eating

Including Over 185 Heart Healthy Nutritious Recipes

Tailored to Your Type

DETAILED CONTENT

CHAPTER 1: INTRODUCTION

In a world where wellness and individuality coexist, the mysterious Blood Type O Diet shines as a beacon of personalized nutrition. Imagine a journey in which your blood type serves as a guiding compass for a healthier, more vibrant self. Step into the world of personalized well-being, where the secrets of the O blood type reveal a distinct story of vitality, strength, and gourmet delight. Join us on an expedition as we explore the tantalizing synthesis of science and flavor, revealing the fascinating story of the Blood Type O Diet! a chapter written in the language of wellness and savored in the brilliant hues of a healthy existence.

UNDERSTANDING THE BLOOD TYPE O DIET

Understanding the Blood Type O Diet is similar to deciphering your unique blueprint for health. Explore the complexities of this nutritional philosophy, in which your blood type serves as a compass, directing you on a personalized path to peak health. Investigate the science behind it, uncovering the mysteries of how Blood Type O people thrive on a precise combination of proteins, veggies, and unusual food choices. It's not just a diet; it's a lifestyle designed to work with your body's natural design. Join the adventure to uncover the mysteries and intricacies of the Blood Type O Diet, where information becomes empowerment for a healthier and more vibrant self.

KITCHEN ESSENTIALS FOR A BLOOD TYPE O DIET

1. Lean Proteins: Stock up on high-quality lean meats such as poultry, fish, and lamb, which correspond to the protein requirements of Blood Type O persons.
2. Green Vegetables: Stock your refrigerator with nutrient-dense greens like kale, spinach, and broccoli, which provide critical vitamins and minerals for good health.
3. Beneficial Fruits: Include fruits such as berries, plums, and figs in your diet to complement your Blood Type O profile.
4. Healthy Oils: Choose beneficial oils such as olive oil or flaxseed oil to help maintain the proper fat balance in your diet.

5. Seafood Selections: Include omega-3 fatty acid-rich seafood, such as salmon and mackerel, to promote heart health and vigor.
6. Nuts and Seeds: Keep a variety of nuts and seeds on hand, including walnuts, pumpkin seeds, and flaxseeds, for a nutritious snack that is appropriate for your blood type.
7. Herbs and Spices: Use blood type-friendly herbs and spices such as ginger, turmeric, and parsley to add flavor as well as potential health advantages to your meals.
8. Avoid: Certain cereals, dairy, and processed foods may not be compatible with the Blood Type O Diet.

MEAL PLANNING TIPS

1. Understand your blood type and related dietary advice. This understanding is the foundation for successful meal planning.
2. Create a weekly menu.
   Plan your meals for the week ahead, including a variety of lean proteins, nutritious vegetables, and fruits appropriate for Blood Type O.
3. Batch cooking allows you to prepare bigger quantities of crucial ingredients, such as proteins and vegetables, to use in multiple meals throughout the week.
4. Rotate between lean protein sources to guarantee a diverse range of nutrients. This could contain chicken, fish, and lamb.
5. Keep blood type-friendly snacks such as nuts, seeds, and fruits on hand to satisfy cravings between meals.
6. Make prudent carb choices by focusing on healthy grains and avoiding those that may not be compatible with the Blood Type O diet.
7. Experiment with Flavors: Use blood type-friendly herbs and spices to increase flavour without sacrificing nutritious value.
8. Remember to drink plenty of water. Stay hydrated throughout the day to promote overall health.
9. Preparing dish components ahead of time on weekends can help simplify weeknight cooking.
10. Listen to your body.
   Pay attention to how your body reacts to various foods. Adjust your food plan according to your energy level, digestion, and overall health.

CHAPTER 2: BREAKFAST DELIGHTS

Omelet with Spinach and Turkey:

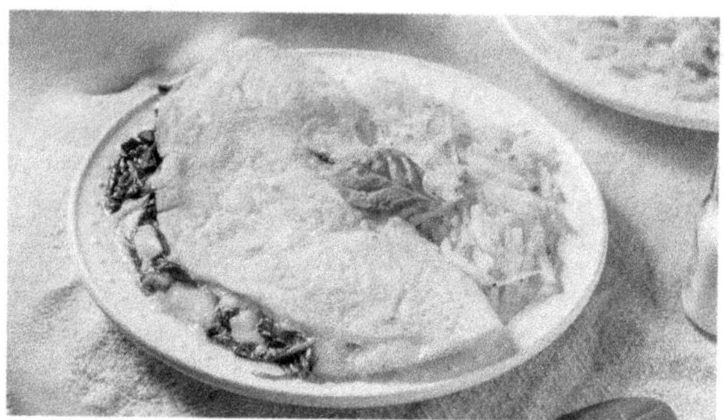

Ingredients:

- 2 Good Eggs
- Nicely cooked, diced or shredded 1/4 Cup cooked Turkey
- Newly harvested spinach leaves 1/2, Cut into pieces
- 2 Tbsp of cubed onion
- 2 Tbsp of Cubed bell pepper
- Cubed cheese 1/4 cup
- 1 Tbsp olive oil
- Pepper and salt to savor

Directions of use:

1. Begin by Dicing the Onion, Bell pepper, Turkey and spinach.
2. Whisk the Eggs together in a bowl until the whites and the Yolks are fully combined, spices the eggs with pepper and pinch of salt to savor.
3. Temperate the olive oil in a non-stick skillet over high temperature, put the cubed onion and bell pepper to the Skillet and grill for about 3 minutes until they begin to soften.

4. Put the Diced spinach into the skillet with the grilled bell pepper and onion, grill for Extra 2 minutes, allowing the spinach to become tender and wilt.

5. Put the Cubed Turkey to the Skillet with the Grilled vegetables, add the whisked eggs over the Turkey and vegetables.

6. Permit the omelet to grill until the edge starts to set.

7. (Optional) sprinkle the diced cheese over half of the omelet.

8. (If using) Carefully turn the other half of the omelet over the cheese to get a round shape.

9. Grill the omelet for an additional 3mins, until the eggs and the cheese have melted (if added).

10. Slide the Omelet in a plate, garnish with an extra diced spinach or herbs (if desired), you can add additional pepper and salt to savor.

11. Dish your spinach and Turkey omelet hot and enjoy a Nutritious meal.

Greek Yogurt with Berries:

Ingredients:

- Plain and Unsweetened Greek yogurt 1/2 cup
- Mixed berries (strawberries,blackberries or blueberries) 1/2 cup
- (If desired) 1 Tbsp of honey
- (If desired) pure vanilla extract 1/4 Tbsp
- A sprinkle of Diced Almonds or walnut

Direction of use:

1. Begin by strawberries, wash and slice properly, If not, clean the other berries and dry gently with a paper towel.

2. (Optional) stir the Greek yogurt with honey and vanilla extract in a small bowl, modify the sweetness to your savor by adding more or less honey.

3. Spoon the sweetened Greek yogurt in a serving bowl or glass.

4. Add mixed berries to the yogurt, you can spread them on top or arrange them neatly.

5. (If desired), Spread a small amount of cubed nuts over the berries for added crunch or savor.

6. Your Greek yogurt with Berries is ready, serve as healthy and delicious delicacies for breakfast.

Quinoa Porridge:

Ingredients:

- Wash thoroughly 1/2 cup quinoa
- 1 cup of water
- 1 cup of preferred milk (such as almond milk, coconut milk depending on your dietary)
- Honey or maple syrup 1 Tbsp
- Ground cinnamon 1/2 Tbsp
- Vanilla extract 1/2 Tbsp
- Pinch of salt
- (Optional) Fresh berries, Sliced bananas or other fruit for topping
- Cubed nuts or seeds for Dress

Direction of Use:

1. Place the Quinoa in a Strainer and wash thoroughly to remove bitterness.

2. In a medium saucepan, Add the rinsed Quinoa with water (1 cup), Permit it to boil over medium-high heat.

3. Reduce the temperature to low, Cover the saucepan, and simmer for about 20 minutes or until quinoa is grilled and most of the liquid is absorbed, the Quinoa should be tender with a slight crunch.

4. Stir in your preferred milk (almond milk or coconut milk) along with honey or maple syrup, ground cinnamon (if using), Vanilla extract (if using) and a pinch of salt.

5. Grill the mixture over low temperature, uncovered, stirring for an additional 5-7 minutes, this will help the porridge to thicken and absorb the savors.

6. Pour the Quinoa porridge into serving bowls, Top with Fresh berries, sliced bananas, or other fruit (if desired), You can also garnish with chopped nuts or seeds for added nutrition.

7. Your homemade Quinoa porridge is now ready to be enjoyed as a wholesome and satisfying breakfast.

Scrambled Eggs with Vegetables:

Ingredients:

- 2 Big eggs
- Cubed bell peppers 1/4 cup
- Cubed onion 1/4 cup
- Cubed tomatoes 1/4 cup
- Cubed spinach or kale 1/4 cup
- Olive oil or ghee 1 Tbsp
- Salt and pepper to savor
- (If desired) a sprinkle of cubed cheese

Direction of use:

1. Prepare the vegetables: cubed the bell peppers, tomatoes and onion, Kale (if desired) remove the tough stems and cut the leaves into small pieces.

2. Crack the eggs and whisk them together in a bowl until the whites and yolks are fully combined, Season the eggs with a pinch of salt and pepper to savor.

3. Grill the vegetables, temperate the ghee or olive oil in a non-stick skillet over medium heat, Add the cubed onion and bell peppers to the skillet and grill for about 2-3 minutes until they start to soften.

4. Add the cubed tomatoes and cubed spinach or kale to the skillet with the grilled onion and bell pepper, Grill for an additional 1-2 minutes until the greens are wilted and tomatoes are slightly softened.
5. Pour the whisked eggs evenly over the grilled vegetables.
6. Using a spatula, gently scramble the eggs and vegetables together, stirring occasionally to ensure even cooking.
7. Add cheese (if desired) sprinkle the diced cheese evenly over the scrambled eggs and vegetables, Allow it to melt into the mixture.
8. Continue to grill and stir the mixture until the eggs are fully grilled and reach your desired level of doneness, They should be slightly creamy and soft.
9. Transfer the scrambled eggs with vegetables to a plate and season with additional salt and pepper (if desired).
10. Serve your delicious and Nutritious scramble hot and enjoy a wholesome breakfast.

Smoked Salmon and Avocado:

Ingredients:

- Smoked salmon 4 pieces
- 1 good ripe avocado
- 1 Good lemon For zest and juice
- Fresh fill 2 Teaspoons, Chopped (if desired)
- Salt and pepper to savor
- Garnishes (optional), capers, Sliced red onion, or microgreens

Direction to use:

1. Slice the ripe avocado into half and remove the pit. Dip out the flesh and place in a bowl.
2. Mash the avocado gently with a fork until it got to your preferable consistency. Make it smoother or slightly chunky, depending on your preference.

3. Squeeze the juice of half a lemon over the mashed avocado. Be aware of catching any seeds. You can add additional Zest for extra flavor. Mix well with the smashed avocado.

4. Season the mixed avocado with a pinch of salt and a dash of freshly ground black pepper. Taste and adjust the seasoning (if necessary)

5. (If desired) mix in the chopped fresh dill to add a burst of fresh herb savor to the avocado.

6. Bring out the pieces of smoked salmon on a serving platter.

7. Scoop the seasoned mashed avocado onto each slice of smoked, sprinkle it gently.

8. Garnish your smoked salmon and avocado with capers, diced red onion, or spread of microgreens (if desired). These add extra savor to the dish.

9. Your smoked salmon and avocado is ready to be served.

Turkey and Veggie Wrap:

Ingredients:

- 1 large whole-grain tortilla
- 4-6 slices of roasted turkey breast
- 1/4 cup hummus
- 1/2 cup mixed salad greens (lettuce, spinach, or your choice)
- 1/4 cup cucumber, thinly sliced
- 1/4 cup cherry tomatoes, halved
- 1/4 cup red bell pepper, thinly sliced
- 1/4 cup shredded carrots
- 1 tablespoon feta cheese, crumbled (optional)
- Salt and pepper to taste

Instructions:

1. Lay the whole-grain tortilla on a clean surface or a large plate.

2. Spread a layer of hummus evenly over the tortilla, leaving a small border around the edges.

3. Arrange the slices of roasted turkey breast in the center of the tortilla.

4. Sprinkle the mixed salad greens over the turkey.

5. Add the cucumber slices, cherry tomatoes, red bell pepper, and shredded carrots on top of the greens.

6. If desired, sprinkle crumbled feta cheese over the vegetables for extra flavor.

7. Season with salt and pepper to taste.

8. Fold the sides of the tortilla towards the center, covering the filling.

9. Starting from the bottom, roll the tortilla tightly to form a wrap.

10. Slice the wrap in half diagonally for easier handling.

11. Serve immediately and enjoy your delicious Turkey and Veggie Wrap!

Peanut Butter and Banana Smoothie:

Ingredients:

- 1 ripe banana, peeled and sliced
- 2 tablespoons peanut butter (smooth or crunchy)
- 1 cup milk (dairy or plant-based)
- 1/2 cup plain yogurt
- 1 tablespoon honey or maple syrup (optional, for sweetness)
- 1/2 teaspoon vanilla extract
- 1 cup ice cubes

Instructions:

1. Place the sliced banana, peanut butter, milk, plain yogurt, honey or maple syrup (if using), vanilla extract, and ice cubes in a blender.

2. Blend on high speed until all the ingredients are well combined and the mixture is smooth.

3. Stop and scrape down the sides of the blender if needed, then blend again to ensure a creamy consistency.

4. Taste the smoothie and adjust sweetness if necessary by adding more honey or maple syrup.

5. Once the desired consistency and sweetness are achieved, pour the smoothie into a glass.

6. Optional: Garnish with a banana slice or a sprinkle of crushed peanuts for texture.

7. Serve immediately and enjoy your nutritious and delicious Peanut Butter and Banana Smoothie!

Breakfast Bowl:

Ingredients:

- 1/2 cup cooked quinoa or oats
- 1/2 cup Greek yogurt (or yogurt of your choice)
- 1/2 cup mixed berries (strawberries, blueberries, raspberries)
- 1 banana, sliced
- 1 tablespoon chia seeds
- 1 tablespoon honey or maple syrup
- 1/4 cup granola
- A sprinkle of nuts (almonds, walnuts, or your preference)
- Optional: A drizzle of nut butter (like almond or peanut butter)

Instructions:

1. Start by cooking quinoa or oats according to package instructions. Let it cool slightly.

2. In a bowl, layer the cooked quinoa or oats.

3. Add a layer of Greek yogurt on top of the quinoa or oats.

4. Arrange the mixed berries and sliced banana over the yogurt.

5. Sprinkle chia seeds evenly over the fruits.

6. Drizzle honey or maple syrup over the entire bowl for sweetness.

7. Top with granola and your choice of nuts for crunch.

8. Optional: Finish with a drizzle of nut butter for added flavor.

9. Mix everything together just before eating to combine the flavors and textures.

10. Enjoy your nutritious and satisfying Breakfast Bowl!

Steel-Cut Oatmeal with Almonds:

Ingredients:

- 1 cup steel-cut oats
- 3 cups water
- 1 cup milk (dairy or plant-based)
- 1/4 teaspoon salt
- 1/2 teaspoon vanilla extract
- 1/4 cup sliced almonds
- 1-2 tablespoons honey or maple syrup (optional, for sweetness)
- Fresh berries or sliced banana for topping (optional)

Instructions:

1. In a medium-sized saucepan, bring 3 cups of water to a boil.
2. Stir in the steel-cut oats and reduce the heat to a low simmer.
3. Add salt and simmer uncovered, stirring occasionally, for about 20-25 minutes or until the oats are creamy and tender.
4. In the last few minutes of cooking, stir in the milk and vanilla extract. Continue to simmer until the oats reach your desired consistency.
5. While the oats are cooking, toast the sliced almonds in a dry skillet over medium heat until they become golden and fragrant. Keep an eye on them to prevent burning.
6. Once the oats are cooked, remove the saucepan from the heat.
7. If desired, sweeten the oatmeal with honey or maple syrup, adjusting to your taste preference.
8. Serve the steel-cut oatmeal in bowls, topped with toasted almonds.
9. Optional: Garnish with fresh berries or sliced banana for added freshness and sweetness.
10. Enjoy your hearty and nutritious Steel-Cut Oatmeal with Almonds!

Fruit Salad with Nuts:

Ingredients:

- 2 cups mixed fresh fruits (such as strawberries, blueberries, grapes, pineapple, and melon), washed and diced
- 1/4 cup chopped nuts (walnuts, almonds, or a mix)
- 2 tablespoons honey or maple syrup
- 1 tablespoon fresh lime or lemon juice
- 1 teaspoon mint leaves, finely chopped (optional)

Instructions:

1. In a large mixing bowl, combine the diced mixed fruits.
2. In a separate small bowl, whisk together honey or maple syrup and lime or lemon juice to create the dressing.
3. Pour the dressing over the mixed fruits and gently toss until all the fruits are coated.
4. Sprinkle the chopped nuts over the fruit mixture.
5. If using, add finely chopped mint leaves for a refreshing touch.
6. Toss the fruit salad gently again to distribute the nuts and mint evenly.
7. Allow the fruit salad to chill in the refrigerator for about 15-30 minutes to let the flavors meld.
8. Just before serving, give the fruit salad a final gentle toss.
9. Serve in individual bowls or as a side dish for a refreshing and nutritious treat.
10. Enjoy your vibrant and delicious Fruit Salad with Nuts!

Tofu Scramble:

Ingredients:

- 1 block (about 14 ounces) firm tofu, pressed and crumbled
- 1 tablespoon olive oil
- 1/2 onion, finely chopped
- 1 bell pepper, diced

- 1 cup spinach or kale, chopped
- 2 cloves garlic, minced
- 1 teaspoon ground turmeric
- 1/2 teaspoon cumin
- 1/2 teaspoon paprika
- Salt and pepper, to taste
- Optional toppings: avocado slices, salsa, nutritional yeast, or fresh herbs

Instructions:

1. Press the tofu to remove excess water by placing it between paper towels or using a tofu press. Crumble the tofu into small pieces.
2. In a large skillet, heat olive oil over medium heat.
3. Add chopped onion and sauté until translucent.
4. Add diced bell pepper and continue to cook until softened.
5. Stir in minced garlic and cook for an additional 1-2 minutes until fragrant.
6. Add the crumbled tofu to the skillet, distributing it evenly.
7. Sprinkle ground turmeric, cumin, paprika, salt, and pepper over the tofu. Stir well to coat the tofu evenly and achieve a yellow color from the turmeric.
8. Add chopped spinach or kale to the skillet and cook until wilted.
9. Continue cooking the tofu mixture for about 5-7 minutes, stirring occasionally, until heated through and slightly crispy.
10. Adjust seasoning to taste.
11. Serve the tofu scramble hot, with optional toppings like avocado slices, salsa, nutritional yeast, or fresh herbs.
12. Enjoy your flavorful and protein-packed Tofu Scramble!

Turkey Sausage with Sweet Potato Hash

Ingredients:

- 1 lb turkey sausage, casings removed
- 2 medium sweet potatoes, peeled and diced

- 1 red bell pepper, diced
- 1 yellow onion, finely chopped
- 2 cloves garlic, minced
- 2 tablespoons olive oil
- 1 teaspoon smoked paprika
- 1/2 teaspoon dried thyme
- Salt and pepper, to taste
- Fresh parsley, chopped (for garnish, optional)
- Fried or poached eggs (optional, for serving)

Instructions:

1. In a large skillet, heat olive oil over medium heat.
2. Add the turkey sausage, breaking it up with a spatula, and cook until browned and cooked through.
3. Remove the cooked turkey sausage from the skillet and set it aside.
4. In the same skillet, add a bit more olive oil if needed. Add the diced sweet potatoes, red bell pepper, and chopped onion.
5. Cook the vegetables over medium heat, stirring occasionally, until the sweet potatoes are tender and slightly crispy on the edges.
6. Add minced garlic to the sweet potato mixture and cook for an additional 1-2 minutes until fragrant.
7. Return the cooked turkey sausage to the skillet with the sweet potatoes and vegetables.
8. Sprinkle smoked paprika, dried thyme, salt, and pepper over the mixture. Stir well to combine.
9. Continue cooking for a few more minutes, allowing the flavors to meld.
10. Optional: Top with fresh chopped parsley for added freshness.
11. Serve the Turkey Sausage with Sweet Potato Hash hot.
12. Optional: Serve with fried or poached eggs on top for a complete and satisfying meal.

CHAPTER 3: LUNCH DELIGHTS

Grilled Chicken Salad:

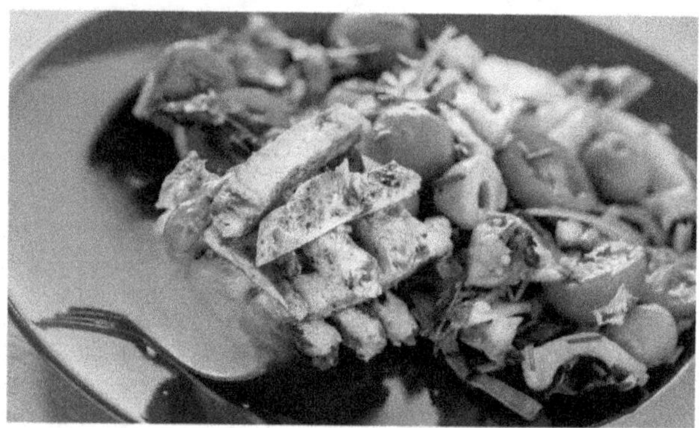

Ingredients:

For the Grilled Chicken:

- 2 boneless, skinless chicken breasts
- 2 tablespoons olive oil
- 1 teaspoon dried oregano
- 1 teaspoon garlic powder
- Salt and pepper, to taste
- Juice of 1 lemon

For the Salad:

- 6 cups mixed salad greens (lettuce, spinach, arugula, etc.)
- 1 cup cherry tomatoes, halved
- 1 cucumber, sliced
- 1 red bell pepper, sliced
- 1/4 red onion, thinly sliced
- 1/2 cup feta cheese, crumbled
- 1/4 cup Kalamata olives, pitted

- 1/4 cup fresh basil leaves, torn

For the Dressing:

- 3 tablespoons olive oil
- 1 tablespoon balsamic vinegar
- 1 teaspoon Dijon mustard
- 1 clove garlic, minced
- Salt and pepper, to taste

Instructions:

For the Grilled Chicken:

1. In a bowl, mix olive oil, dried oregano, garlic powder, salt, and pepper. Add lemon juice and stir well.
2. Place the chicken breasts in a resealable plastic bag or shallow dish. Pour the marinade over the chicken, making sure it's well-coated. Marinate for at least 30 minutes, or refrigerate for up to 24 hours.
3. Preheat the grill or grill pan over medium-high heat. Grill the chicken for about 6-7 minutes per side or until cooked through with an internal temperature of 165°F (74°C).
4. Allow the grilled chicken to rest for a few minutes before slicing it into strips.

For the Salad:

5. In a large salad bowl, combine mixed greens, cherry tomatoes, cucumber, red bell pepper, red onion, feta cheese, Kalamata olives, and torn basil leaves.

For the Dressing:

6. In a small bowl, whisk together olive oil, balsamic vinegar, Dijon mustard, minced garlic, salt, and pepper.
7. Drizzle the dressing over the salad and toss gently to combine.
8. Top the salad with grilled chicken strips.
9. Serve immediately and enjoy your fresh and flavorful Grilled Chicken Salad!

Lentil Soup:

Ingredients:

- 1 cup dried green or brown lentils, rinsed and picked over
- 1 onion, finely chopped
- 2 carrots, peeled and diced
- 2 celery stalks, diced
- 3 cloves garlic, minced
- 1 can (14 oz) diced tomatoes
- 6 cups vegetable or chicken broth
- 1 teaspoon ground cumin
- 1 teaspoon ground coriander
- 1/2 teaspoon smoked paprika
- 1 bay leaf
- Salt and pepper, to taste
- 2 tablespoons olive oil
- Juice of 1 lemon (optional, for serving)
- Fresh parsley, chopped (for garnish, optional)

Instructions:

1. In a large pot, heat olive oil over medium heat. Add chopped onions, carrots, and celery. Sauté until the vegetables are softened, about 5 minutes.
2. Add minced garlic and sauté for an additional 1-2 minutes until fragrant.
3. Rinse the lentils under cold water and add them to the pot.
4. Pour in the diced tomatoes with their juice and stir to combine.
5. Add vegetable or chicken broth, ground cumin, ground coriander, smoked paprika, bay leaf, salt, and pepper. Stir well.
6. Bring the soup to a boil, then reduce the heat to low. Cover and simmer for about 25-30 minutes or until the lentils are tender.
7. Taste and adjust the seasoning if needed.
8. Optional: Stir in the lemon juice for a fresh citrusy flavor.

9. Remove the bay leaf before serving.

10. Ladle the lentil soup into bowls, garnish with fresh parsley if desired, and serve hot.

Quinoa and Vegetable Stir-Fry:

Ingredients:

- 1 cup quinoa, rinsed and drained
- 2 cups water
- 2 tablespoons soy sauce
- 1 tablespoon sesame oil
- 1 tablespoon olive oil
- 2 cloves garlic, minced
- 1 tablespoon ginger, grated
- 1 medium carrot, julienned
- 1 bell pepper, thinly sliced (any color)
- 1 zucchini, thinly sliced
- 1 cup broccoli florets
- 1 cup snap peas, ends trimmed
- 2 green onions, chopped
- Sesame seeds for garnish (optional)

Instructions:

1. In a medium saucepan, combine quinoa and water. Bring to a boil, then reduce heat to low, cover, and simmer for 15-20 minutes or until the quinoa is cooked and water is absorbed.
2. While the quinoa is cooking, prepare the vegetables.
3. In a small bowl, mix soy sauce and sesame oil. Set aside.
4. Heat olive oil in a large wok or skillet over medium-high heat.
5. Add minced garlic and grated ginger, sautéing for about 1 minute until fragrant.

6. Add julienned carrots, sliced bell pepper, zucchini, broccoli florets, and snap peas to the wok. Stir-fry for 5-7 minutes or until the vegetables are crisp-tender.

7. Once the vegetables are cooked, add the cooked quinoa to the wok.

8. Pour the soy sauce and sesame oil mixture over the quinoa and vegetables. Stir well to combine.

9. Cook for an additional 2-3 minutes, allowing the flavors to meld.

10. Adjust seasoning if needed and stir in chopped green onions.

11. Optional: Garnish with sesame seeds for added texture.

Turkey Lettuce Wraps:

Ingredients:

For the Turkey Filling:

- 1 lb ground turkey
- 1 tablespoon olive oil
- 1 onion, finely chopped
- 2 cloves garlic, minced
- 1 tablespoon soy sauce
- 1 tablespoon hoisin sauce
- 1 teaspoon ginger, grated
- 1 cup water chestnuts, finely chopped
- 2 green onions, chopped
- Salt and pepper, to taste

For Assembling:

- Large iceberg or butter lettuce leaves, washed and patted dry
- Sriracha or hot sauce (optional, for serving)
- Additional hoisin sauce (for drizzling, optional)
- Chopped cilantro or mint (for garnish, optional)

Instructions:

1. In a large skillet, heat olive oil over medium-high heat.

2. Add chopped onion and cook until softened, about 2-3 minutes.

3. Add minced garlic and grated ginger, sautéing for an additional 1-2 minutes until fragrant.

4. Add ground turkey to the skillet, breaking it up with a spatula. Cook until browned and cooked through.

5. Stir in soy sauce and hoisin sauce, ensuring the turkey is well-coated.

6. Add chopped water chestnuts and cook for an additional 2-3 minutes.

7. Season with salt and pepper to taste.

8. Remove the skillet from heat and stir in chopped green onions.

9. Arrange the large lettuce leaves on a serving platter.

10. Spoon the turkey mixture onto each lettuce leaf, creating wraps.

11. Optional: Drizzle additional hoisin sauce on top for extra flavor.

12. Garnish with chopped cilantro or mint if desired.

13. Serve immediately with Sriracha or hot sauce on the side.

Salmon with Steamed Broccoli:

Ingredients:

- 4 salmon fillets (about 6 oz each), skin-on or skinless
- Salt and pepper, to taste
- 1 tablespoon olive oil
- 1 teaspoon lemon zest
- 1 tablespoon lemon juice
- 2 cloves garlic, minced
- 1 teaspoon Dijon mustard
- 1 tablespoon fresh dill, chopped (or 1 teaspoon dried dill)
- 1 bunch broccoli, cut into florets
- Lemon wedges, for serving

Instructions:

1. Preheat the oven to 400°F (200°C).

2. Season the salmon fillets with salt and pepper on both sides.

3. In a small bowl, mix together olive oil, lemon zest, lemon juice, minced garlic, Dijon mustard, and chopped dill to create the marinade.

4. Place the salmon fillets in a shallow dish and brush them with the marinade, ensuring they are well-coated. Let them marinate for about 15 minutes.

5. While the salmon is marinating, prepare the broccoli by cutting it into florets.

6. Place broccoli florets in a steamer basket over boiling water. Steam for about 5-7 minutes or until they are tender-crisp.

7. Heat a large oven-safe skillet over medium-high heat. Add a bit of olive oil if needed.

8. Place the marinated salmon fillets in the skillet, skin-side down if they have skin.

9. Sear the salmon for 2-3 minutes on each side until a golden crust forms.

10. Transfer the skillet to the preheated oven and bake for about 8-10 minutes or until the salmon is cooked through and flakes easily with a fork.

11. Serve the salmon on a plate alongside steamed broccoli.

12. Optional: Garnish with additional fresh dill and serve with lemon wedges.

Bison Burger:

Ingredients:

- 1 lb ground bison meat
- 1 tablespoon olive oil
- 1/2 teaspoon garlic powder
- 1/2 teaspoon onion powder
- 1 teaspoon dried oregano
- Salt and pepper to taste
- 4 whole grain or brioche burger buns
- Lettuce, tomato, red onion, and other toppings of choice
- Cheese slices (optional)
- Condiments (ketchup, mustard, mayo etc.)

Instructions:

1. Preheat the grill or stovetop grilling pan over medium-high heat.
2. In a bowl, gently mix the ground bison meat with olive oil, garlic powder, onion powder, dried oregano, salt, and pepper. Avoid over-mixing to keep the meat tender.
3. Divide the seasoned bison meat into four equal portions and shape them into burger patties.
4. Place the burger patties on the preheated grill or grilling pan.
5. Cook the bison burgers for approximately 4-5 minutes per side, or until they reach your desired level of doneness. Bison is lean meat, so be cautious not to overcook to maintain juiciness.
6. Optional: Add cheese slices to the burgers during the last minute of cooking to melt.
7. While the burgers are cooking, toast the burger buns on the grill or in a toaster.
8. Assemble the burgers by placing each cooked bison patty on a toasted bun.
9. Top with lettuce, tomato slices, red onion, and any other desired toppings.
10. Add condiments of choice—ketchup, mustard, mayo—or your preferred sauce.
11. Place the top bun on each burger to complete.
12. Serve the Bison Burgers hot, and enjoy your lean and flavorful burger!

Tuna Salad:

Ingredients:

- 2 cans (5 oz each) canned tuna, drained
- 1/2 cup celery, finely chopped
- 1/4 cup red onion, finely chopped
- 1/4 cup dill pickles, finely chopped
- 1/4 cup mayonnaise
- 1 tablespoon Dijon mustard
- 1 tablespoon lemon juice

- Salt and pepper, to taste
- Optional: 1/4 cup fresh parsley, chopped
- Optional: Lettuce leaves or whole-grain bread for serving

Instructions:

1. In a large mixing bowl, flake the drained tuna with a fork.
2. Add finely chopped celery, red onion, and dill pickles to the bowl.
3. In a separate small bowl, mix together mayonnaise, Dijon mustard, and lemon juice.
4. Pour the mayo-mustard mixture over the tuna and vegetables. Stir well to combine.
5. Season the tuna salad with salt and pepper to taste. Adjust the seasoning according to your preference.
6. Optional: Fold in chopped fresh parsley for added freshness and flavor.
7. Refrigerate the tuna salad for at least 30 minutes before serving to allow the flavors to meld.
8. Serve the tuna salad on a bed of lettuce leaves, as a sandwich filling, or with whole-grain bread.

Sushi Rolls:

Ingredients:

For Sushi Rice:

- 2 cups sushi rice
- 2 1/2 cups water
- 1/2 cup rice vinegar
- 3 tablespoons sugar
- 1 teaspoon salt

For Sushi Filling:

- Nori (seaweed) sheets
- Fresh fish (salmon, tuna), thinly sliced

- Vegetables (cucumber, avocado, carrot), julienned
- Crab or imitation crab sticks
- Sesame seeds (optional)

For Rolling:

- Bamboo sushi rolling mat
- Plastic wrap (to cover the bamboo mat)
- Soy sauce, for dipping
- Pickled ginger and wasabi, for serving

Instructions:

Prepare Sushi Rice:

1. Rinse sushi rice under cold water until the water runs clear.
2. Combine rice and water in a rice cooker and cook according to the manufacturer's instructions.
3. In a small saucepan, heat rice vinegar, sugar, and salt over low heat until the sugar and salt dissolve.
4. Once the rice is cooked, transfer it to a large bowl and gently fold in the vinegar mixture. Allow the rice to cool to room temperature.

Prepare Sushi Filling:

5. Lay a sheet of nori, shiny side down, on the bamboo rolling mat covered with plastic wrap.
6. Moisten your hands with water to prevent the rice from sticking. Spread a thin layer of sushi rice evenly over the nori, leaving a small border at the top.
7. Arrange your desired fillings (fish, vegetables, crab sticks) horizontally along the bottom edge of the rice.
8. Optional: Sprinkle sesame seeds over the fillings for added texture.

Rolling the Sushi:

9. Using the bamboo mat, lift the bottom edge of the nori and rice over the fillings, then continue to roll tightly until you reach the top border.
10. Wet the top border with a bit of water to seal the sushi roll.

11. Place the rolled sushi seam-side down on a cutting board.

12. Using a sharp, wet knife, slice the sushi roll into bite-sized pieces.

Turkey and Avocado Wrap:

Ingredients:

- 1 large whole-grain or spinach tortilla
- 4-6 slices of roasted turkey breast
- 1/2 ripe avocado, sliced
- 1/4 cup cherry tomatoes, halved
- 1/4 cup cucumber, thinly sliced
- 1/4 cup red onion, thinly sliced
- 1/2 cup mixed salad greens (lettuce, spinach, arugula)
- 1 tablespoon mayonnaise or Greek yogurt (optional)
- 1 teaspoon Dijon mustard (optional)
- Salt and pepper, to taste

Instructions:

1. Lay the tortilla on a clean surface or a large plate.
2. If using, spread a thin layer of mayonnaise or Greek yogurt over the tortilla, leaving a small border around the edges.
3. Place the slices of roasted turkey breast in the center of the tortilla.
4. Arrange avocado slices, cherry tomatoes, cucumber, red onion, and mixed salad greens on top of the turkey.
5. Optional: Drizzle Dijon mustard over the ingredients for added flavor.
6. Season with salt and pepper to taste.
7. Fold the sides of the tortilla towards the center, covering the filling.
8. Starting from the bottom, roll the tortilla tightly to form a wrap.
9. Slice the wrap in half diagonally for easier handling.
10. Secure with toothpicks if needed.
11. Serve immediately and enjoy your Turkey and Avocado Wrap!

Chicken and Vegetable Stir-Fry:

Ingredients:

- 1 lb boneless, skinless chicken breasts, thinly sliced
- 2 tablespoons soy sauce
- 1 tablespoon oyster sauce
- 1 tablespoon hoisin sauce
- 1 tablespoon cornstarch
- 2 tablespoons vegetable oil, divided
- 1 onion, thinly sliced
- 2 bell peppers (any color), thinly sliced
- 1 cup broccoli florets
- 1 carrot, julienned
- 2 cloves garlic, minced
- 1 teaspoon ginger, grated
- 2 green onions, chopped (for garnish)
- Sesame seeds (for garnish, optional)
- Cooked rice or noodles, for serving

Instructions:

1. In a bowl, mix soy sauce, oyster sauce, hoisin sauce, and cornstarch. Add sliced chicken and toss to coat. Let it marinate for about 15-20 minutes.
2. Heat 1 tablespoon of vegetable oil in a wok or large skillet over high heat.
3. Add the marinated chicken and stir-fry until it's browned and cooked through. Remove the chicken from the wok and set aside.
4. In the same wok, add another tablespoon of oil.
5. Stir in minced garlic and grated ginger, sautéing for about 30 seconds until fragrant.
6. Add sliced onion, bell peppers, broccoli florets, and julienned carrot. Stir-fry for 3-4 minutes or until the vegetables are crisp-tender.
7. Return the cooked chicken to the wok, tossing to combine with the vegetables.

8. Stir-fry for an additional 2-3 minutes to heat through.

9. Optional: Drizzle a bit more soy sauce or hoisin sauce for extra flavor.

10. Sprinkle chopped green onions and sesame seeds over the stir-fry for garnish.

11. Serve the Chicken and Vegetable Stir-Fry over cooked rice or noodles.

Lentil and Vegetable Salad:

Ingredients:

For the Salad:

- 1 cup dried green or brown lentils, rinsed
- 3 cups water
- 1 cup cherry tomatoes, halved
- 1 cucumber, diced
- 1 red bell pepper, diced
- 1/4 cup red onion, finely chopped
- 1/4 cup fresh parsley, chopped
- 1/4 cup feta cheese, crumbled (optional)
- Salt and pepper, to taste

For the Dressing:

- 3 tablespoons olive oil
- 2 tablespoons balsamic vinegar
- 1 teaspoon Dijon mustard
- 1 clove garlic, minced
- Salt and pepper, to taste

Instructions:

1. In a medium saucepan, combine lentils and water. Bring to a boil, then reduce heat to low, cover, and simmer for 20-25 minutes or until lentils are tender but still hold their shape. Drain any excess water and let them cool.

2. In a large bowl, combine the cooked lentils, cherry tomatoes, cucumber, red bell pepper, red onion, and fresh parsley.

3. Optional: Add crumbled feta cheese for an extra burst of flavor.

4. In a small bowl, whisk together olive oil, balsamic vinegar, Dijon mustard, minced garlic, salt, and pepper to create the dressing.

5. Pour the dressing over the lentil and vegetable mixture. Toss gently to coat everything evenly.

6. Taste and adjust the seasoning if needed.

7. Chill the Lentil and Vegetable Salad in the refrigerator for at least 30 minutes to allow the flavors to meld.
8. Before serving, give the salad a final gentle toss.

Beef and Broccoli Stir-Fry:

Ingredients:
- 1 lb flank steak or sirloin, thinly sliced against the grain
- 3 cups broccoli florets
- 3 tablespoons soy sauce
- 2 tablespoons oyster sauce
- 1 tablespoon hoisin sauce
- 1 tablespoon cornstarch
- 1 tablespoon sesame oil
- 2 tablespoons vegetable oil, divided
- 3 cloves garlic, minced
- 1 teaspoon ginger, grated
- 1/4 cup water
- Cooked white rice, for serving
- Sesame seeds and chopped green onions (for garnish, optional)

Instructions:
1. In a bowl, combine sliced beef with soy sauce, oyster sauce, hoisin sauce, cornstarch, and sesame oil. Let it marinate for about 15-20 minutes.
2. Heat 1 tablespoon of vegetable oil in a wok or large skillet over high heat.
3. Add the marinated beef and stir-fry for 2-3 minutes or until it's browned and cooked through. Remove the beef from the wok and set aside.
4. In the same wok, add another tablespoon of oil.
5. Stir in minced garlic and grated ginger, sautéing for about 30 seconds until fragrant.
6. Add broccoli florets to the wok and stir-fry for 2-3 minutes or until they are bright green and crisp-tender.
7. Pour in 1/4 cup of water to create steam and help cook the broccoli.
8. Return the cooked beef to the wok and toss everything together.
9. Stir-fry for an additional 1-2 minutes to heat through and allow the flavors to meld.
10. Optional: Drizzle a bit more soy sauce or sesame oil for extra flavor.
11. Serve the Beef and Broccoli Stir-Fry over cooked white rice.

CHAPTER 4: DINNER DELIGHTS

Grilled Salmon:

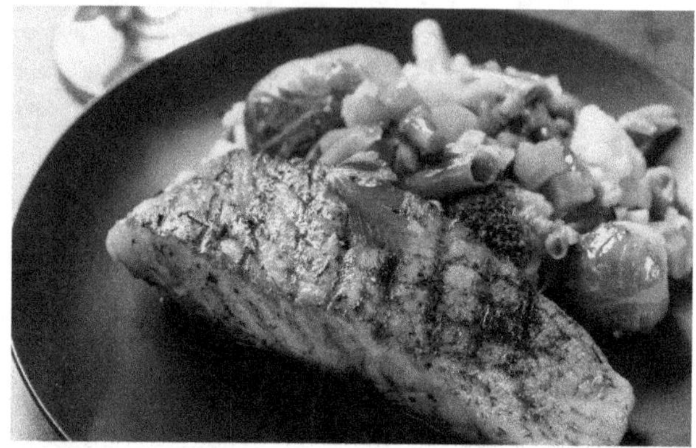

Ingredients:

- 4 salmon fillets (about 6 oz each) skin-on or skinless
- 2 tablespoons olive oil
- 1 tablespoon soy sauce
- 1 tablespoon lemon juice
- 2 cloves garlic, minced
- 1 teaspoon Dijon mustard
- 1 teaspoon honey or maple syrup
- 1 teaspoon dried dill (or 1 tablespoon fresh dill, chopped)
- Salt and pepper, to taste
- Lemon wedges, for serving

Instructions:

1. Preheat the grill to medium-high heat.
2. In a bowl, whisk together olive oil, soy sauce, lemon juice, minced garlic, Dijon mustard, honey or maple syrup, dried dill, salt, and pepper to create the marinade.

3. Place the salmon fillets in a shallow dish and pour half of the marinade over them. Let the salmon marinate for about 15-20 minutes.

4. Reserve the remaining marinade for basting and serving.

5. Brush the grill grates with a bit of oil to prevent sticking.

6. Place the marinated salmon fillets on the preheated grill, skin-side down if they have skin.

7. Grill the salmon for approximately 4-5 minutes per side or until it's cooked through and flakes easily with a fork. Baste the salmon with the reserved marinade during grilling.

8. Optional: For extra grill marks and flavor, you can close the grill lid during cooking.

9. Once cooked, transfer the grilled salmon to a serving platter.

10. Drizzle any remaining marinade over the grilled salmon for added flavor.

11. Serve the Grilled Salmon hot with lemon wedges on the side.

Chicken Stir-Fry:

Ingredients:

- 1 lb boneless, skinless chicken breasts, thinly sliced
- 2 tablespoons soy sauce
- 1 tablespoon oyster sauce
- 1 tablespoon hoisin sauce
- 1 teaspoon sesame oil
- 2 tablespoons vegetable oil
- 1 onion, thinly sliced
- 1 bell pepper, thinly sliced
- 1 cup broccoli florets
- 2 carrots, julienned
- 3 cloves garlic, minced
- 1-inch ginger, grated

- 2 green onions, sliced
- Cooked rice for serving

Instructions:

1. In a bowl, marinate the sliced chicken with soy sauce, oyster sauce, hoisin sauce, and sesame oil. Let it sit for at least 15 minutes.
2. Heat 1 tablespoon of vegetable oil in a wok or large skillet over medium-high heat.
3. Add the marinated chicken to the hot pan and stir-fry until cooked through. Remove from the pan and set aside.
4. In the same pan, add another tablespoon of vegetable oil. Stir in garlic and ginger, sautéing for about 30 seconds until fragrant.
5. Add sliced onions, bell peppers, broccoli, and julienned carrots to the pan. Stir-fry the vegetables until they are crisp-tender, about 3-4 minutes.
6. Return the cooked chicken to the pan, tossing everything together until well combined and heated through.
7. Sprinkle sliced green onions over the stir-fry, and give it a final toss.
8. Serve the chicken stir-fry over cooked rice.

Turkey Chili:

Ingredients:

- 1 lb ground turkey
- 1 tablespoon olive oil
- 1 onion, finely chopped
- 3 cloves garlic, minced
- 1 bell pepper, diced
- 1 jalapeño, seeded and minced (optional for heat)
- 2 cans (15 oz each) kidney beans, drained and rinsed
- 1 can (28 oz) crushed tomatoes
- 1 can (14 oz) diced tomatoes, undrained
- 2 tablespoons tomato paste

- 2 teaspoons chili powder
- 1 teaspoon ground cumin
- 1 teaspoon paprika
- 1/2 teaspoon dried oregano
- Salt and black pepper to taste
- Optional toppings: shredded cheese, sour cream, chopped green onions

Instructions:

1. In a large pot, heat olive oil over medium heat. Add the ground turkey and cook until browned, breaking it apart with a spoon as it cooks.
2. Add chopped onions, minced garlic, diced bell pepper, and minced jalapeño (if using) to the pot. Sauté until the vegetables are softened.
3. Stir in chili powder, ground cumin, paprika, and dried oregano. Cook for 1-2 minutes to allow the spices to become fragrant.
4. Add crushed tomatoes, diced tomatoes (with their juice), tomato paste, and drained kidney beans to the pot. Mix well.
5. Season the chili with salt and black pepper to taste. If you prefer a spicier chili, you can add a bit more chili powder or cayenne pepper at this point.
6. Bring the chili to a simmer, then reduce the heat to low. Cover and let it simmer for at least 30 minutes to allow the flavors to meld.
7. Taste and adjust the seasoning if needed. If the chili is too thick, you can add a bit of water or broth to achieve your desired consistency.
8. Serve the turkey chili hot, topped with shredded cheese, a dollop of sour cream, and chopped green onions if desired.

Bison Steak:

Ingredients:

- 2 bison steaks (about 8 oz each)
- 2 tablespoons olive oil
- 2 cloves garlic, minced

- 1 teaspoon dried thyme
- Salt and black pepper to taste
- Optional: Fresh herbs for garnish (rosemary or parsley)

Instructions:

1. Preheat your grill or stovetop grill pan over medium-high heat.
2. Pat the bison steaks dry with paper towels to remove excess moisture.
3. In a small bowl, mix together olive oil, minced garlic, dried thyme, salt, and black pepper to create a marinade.
4. Brush both sides of the bison steaks with the prepared marinade.
5. Place the steaks on the preheated grill and cook for about 4-5 minutes per side for medium-rare, or adjust the cooking time according to your desired doneness.
6. Allow the bison steaks to rest for a few minutes after cooking to let the juices redistribute.
7. Optionally, garnish with fresh herbs like rosemary or parsley before serving.
8. Slice the bison steaks against the grain and serve immediately.

Shrimp and Vegetable Skewers:

Ingredients:

- 1 lb large shrimp, peeled and deveined
- 1 zucchini, sliced into rounds
- 1 bell pepper, cut into chunks
- 1 red onion, cut into wedges
- Cherry tomatoes
- 2 tablespoons olive oil
- 2 cloves garlic, minced
- 1 teaspoon lemon zest
- 2 tablespoons lemon juice
- 1 teaspoon dried oregano
- Salt and black pepper to taste

- Wooden or metal skewers

Instructions:

1. If using wooden skewers, soak them in water for at least 30 minutes to prevent burning.
2. In a bowl, combine olive oil, minced garlic, lemon zest, lemon juice, dried oregano, salt, and black pepper to create the marinade.
3. Thread the shrimp, zucchini rounds, bell pepper chunks, red onion wedges, and cherry tomatoes onto the skewers, alternating the ingredients.
4. Brush the skewers generously with the prepared marinade, ensuring all the ingredients are coated.
5. Preheat a grill or grill pan to medium-high heat.
6. Place the skewers on the grill and cook for about 2-3 minutes per side, or until the shrimp are opaque and vegetables are tender with a slight char.
7. While grilling, continue to brush the skewers with the marinade for added flavor.
8. Once cooked, remove the skewers from the grill and let them rest for a minute.
9. Serve the shrimp and vegetable skewers hot, garnished with additional lemon wedges if desired.

Baked Cod:

Ingredients:

- 4 cod fillets (about 6 oz each)
- 2 tablespoons olive oil
- 2 tablespoons lemon juice
- 2 cloves garlic, minced
- 1 teaspoon dried thyme
- 1 teaspoon paprika
- Salt and black pepper to taste
- Lemon wedges for serving
- Fresh parsley, chopped (optional, for garnish)

Instructions:

1. Preheat your oven to 400°F (200°C).
2. Pat the cod fillets dry with paper towels and place them in a baking dish.
3. In a small bowl, whisk together olive oil, lemon juice, minced garlic, dried thyme, paprika, salt, and black pepper to create the marinade.
4. Pour the marinade over the cod fillets, ensuring they are well coated. You can let them marinate for about 15-20 minutes for added flavor.
5. Bake the cod in the preheated oven for approximately 15-20 minutes or until the fish is opaque and easily flakes with a fork.
6. If you want a slightly browned top, you can broil the cod for an additional 2-3 minutes at the end of the baking time.
7. Remove the baked cod from the oven and let it rest for a couple of minutes.
8. Serve the cod fillets hot, garnished with fresh parsley if desired, and accompanied by lemon wedges for a burst of citrus flavor.

Lentil Soup:

Ingredients:

- 1 cup dried green or brown lentils, rinsed and drained
- 1 onion, finely chopped
- 2 carrots, diced
- 2 celery stalks, diced
- 3 cloves garlic, minced
- 1 can (14 oz) diced tomatoes, undrained
- 6 cups vegetable or chicken broth
- 1 teaspoon ground cumin
- 1 teaspoon ground coriander
- 1/2 teaspoon smoked paprika
- 1 bay leaf
- Salt and black pepper to taste

- 2 tablespoons olive oil
- Fresh lemon wedges (optional, for serving)
- Fresh parsley, chopped (optional, for garnish)

Instructions:

1. In a large pot, heat olive oil over medium heat. Add chopped onions, carrots, and celery. Sauté until the vegetables are softened, about 5 minutes.
2. Add minced garlic and continue to sauté for an additional 1-2 minutes until fragrant.
3. Stir in ground cumin, ground coriander, and smoked paprika. Cook for another 1-2 minutes to enhance the flavors.
4. Add lentils, diced tomatoes (with their juice), vegetable or chicken broth, and the bay leaf to the pot. Season with salt and black pepper to taste.
5. Bring the soup to a boil, then reduce the heat to low, cover, and simmer for about 25-30 minutes or until the lentils are tender.
6. If the soup is too thick, you can add more broth or water to achieve your desired consistency.
7. Taste and adjust the seasoning if needed. Remove the bay leaf before serving.
8. Ladle the lentil soup into bowls, and garnish with fresh parsley if desired. Serve with lemon wedges on the side for a burst of citrus flavor.

Beef and Broccoli:

Ingredients:

- 1 lb flank steak, thinly sliced
- 1/2 cup low-sodium soy sauce
- 2 tablespoons oyster sauce
- 2 tablespoons hoisin sauce
- 1 tablespoon cornstarch
- 2 tablespoons vegetable oil
- 3 cups broccoli florets

- 3 cloves garlic, minced
- 1 tablespoon fresh ginger, grated
- 2 green onions, sliced
- Cooked white rice for serving
- Sesame seeds for garnish (optional)

Instructions:

1. In a bowl, whisk together soy sauce, oyster sauce, hoisin sauce, and cornstarch to create the marinade.
2. Place the sliced flank steak in the marinade, ensuring it's well-coated. Let it marinate for at least 15 minutes.
3. Heat 1 tablespoon of vegetable oil in a wok or large skillet over medium-high heat.
4. Add the marinated beef to the hot pan and stir-fry until it's browned and cooked to your liking. Remove the beef from the pan and set it aside.
5. In the same pan, add another tablespoon of vegetable oil. Stir in minced garlic and grated ginger, sautéing for about 30 seconds until fragrant.
6. Add broccoli florets to the pan and stir-fry for 2-3 minutes until they are crisp-tender.
7. Return the cooked beef to the pan, tossing everything together until well combined and heated through.
8. Sprinkle sliced green onions over the beef and broccoli, and give it a final toss.
9. Serve the beef and broccoli over cooked white rice, and garnish with sesame seeds if desired.

Turkey and Quinoa Stuffed Peppers:

Ingredients:

- 4 large bell peppers, halved and seeds removed
- 1 cup quinoa, rinsed
- 1 lb ground turkey
- 1 tablespoon olive oil

- 1 onion, finely chopped
- 2 cloves garlic, minced
- 1 can (14 oz) diced tomatoes, drained
- 1 cup black beans, drained and rinsed
- 1 cup corn kernels (fresh, frozen, or canned)
- 1 teaspoon ground cumin
- 1 teaspoon chili powder
- Salt and black pepper to taste
- 1 cup shredded cheese (cheddar, Monterey Jack, or your choice)
- Fresh cilantro, chopped (optional, for garnish)
- Sour cream for serving (optional)

Instructions:

1. Preheat the oven to 375°F (190°C).
2. Cook quinoa according to package instructions. Set aside.
3. Heat olive oil in a large skillet over medium heat. Add chopped onions and garlic, sautéing until softened.
4. Add ground turkey to the skillet and cook until browned, breaking it apart with a spoon as it cooks.
5. Stir in diced tomatoes, black beans, corn, ground cumin, and chili powder. Cook for an additional 3-4 minutes to combine the flavors. Season with salt and black pepper to taste.
6. In a large mixing bowl, combine the cooked quinoa with the turkey mixture.
7. Place the bell pepper halves in a baking dish. Spoon the turkey and quinoa mixture into each pepper half.
8. Sprinkle shredded cheese over the top of each stuffed pepper.
9. Cover the baking dish with foil and bake in the preheated oven for 25-30 minutes or until the peppers are tender.
10. Optionally, remove the foil during the last 5 minutes of baking to allow the cheese to melt and slightly brown.

11. Garnish with chopped cilantro if desired and serve the stuffed peppers hot. Optionally, serve with a dollop of sour cream.

Grilled Portobello Mushrooms:

Ingredients:

- 4 large Portobello mushrooms, stems removed
- 3 tablespoons balsamic vinegar
- 2 tablespoons olive oil
- 2 cloves garlic, minced
- 1 teaspoon dried thyme
- Salt and black pepper to taste
- Fresh parsley, chopped (optional, for garnish)

Instructions:

1. Clean the Portobello mushrooms by gently wiping them with a damp cloth or brushing off any dirt. Remove the stems.
2. In a small bowl, whisk together balsamic vinegar, olive oil, minced garlic, dried thyme, salt, and black pepper to create the marinade.
3. Place the cleaned Portobello mushrooms in a shallow dish, gill side up. Pour the marinade over the mushrooms, ensuring they are well-coated. Let them marinate for at least 15-20 minutes.
4. Preheat your grill to medium-high heat.
5. Place the marinated Portobello mushrooms on the grill, gill side down. Grill for about 4-5 minutes on each side or until they are tender.
6. While grilling, brush the mushrooms with any remaining marinade to enhance the flavor.
7. Once the mushrooms are cooked, remove them from the grill and let them rest for a minute.
8. Optionally, garnish with chopped fresh parsley for added freshness.

9. Serve the grilled Portobello mushrooms as a side dish, on a salad, or as a meaty element in a sandwich.

Baked Chicken Thighs:

Ingredients:

- 4 bone-in, skin-on chicken thighs
- 2 tablespoons olive oil
- 2 teaspoons garlic powder
- 1 teaspoon onion powder
- 1 teaspoon paprika
- 1 teaspoon dried thyme
- 1 teaspoon dried rosemary
- Salt and black pepper to taste
- Fresh parsley, chopped (optional, for garnish)

Instructions:

1. Preheat the oven to 400°F (200°C).
2. Pat the chicken thighs dry with paper towels to remove excess moisture.
3. In a small bowl, mix together olive oil, garlic powder, onion powder, paprika, dried thyme, dried rosemary, salt, and black pepper to create a seasoning blend.
4. Place the chicken thighs in a baking dish, skin side up.
5. Brush the chicken thighs with the prepared seasoning blend, ensuring they are well-coated.
6. Bake in the preheated oven for approximately 35-40 minutes or until the internal temperature reaches 165°F (74°C) and the skin is crispy.
7. If you want the skin to be even crispier, you can broil the chicken thighs for an additional 2-3 minutes at the end of the baking time.
8. Once baked, remove the chicken thighs from the oven and let them rest for a few minutes.
9. Garnish with chopped fresh parsley if desired.

10. Serve the baked chicken thighs hot, paired with your favorite side dishes.

Sushi:

Ingredients:

- 2 cups sushi rice
- 2 1/2 cups water
- 1/2 cup rice vinegar
- 3 tablespoons sugar
- 1 teaspoon salt
- Nori seaweed sheets
- Fresh fish (salmon, tuna), thinly sliced
- Vegetables (cucumber, avocado, carrot), julienned
- Soy sauce, for dipping
- Pickled ginger, for serving
- Wasabi, for serving
- Bamboo sushi rolling mat

Instructions:

For Sushi Rice:

1. Rinse sushi rice under cold water until the water runs clear.
2. Combine rice and water in a rice cooker and cook according to the cooker's instructions.
3. In a small saucepan, heat rice vinegar, sugar, and salt over low heat until sugar dissolves. Let it cool.
4. Once the rice is cooked, transfer it to a large bowl. Gradually add the vinegar mixture, gently folding to combine. Let it cool to room temperature.

For Sushi Rolls:

1. Place a sheet of nori, shiny side down, on the bamboo rolling mat.
2. Wet your hands to prevent sticking, then grab a handful of sushi rice and spread it evenly over the nori, leaving about 1 inch at the top.

3. Arrange thin slices of fish and julienned vegetables along the bottom edge of the rice.

4. Using the bamboo mat, carefully roll the sushi away from you, applying gentle pressure to shape it into a cylinder.

5. Wet the top edge of the nori with a bit of water to seal the roll.

6. With a sharp, damp knife, slice the roll into bite-sized pieces.

7. Repeat the process with different combinations of fish and vegetables.

Serve:

1. Arrange the sushi pieces on a plate.

2. Serve with soy sauce, pickled ginger, and wasabi on the side.

3. Enjoy your homemade sushi rolls!

CHAPTER 5: SATISFYING SNACKS AND APPETIZERS

Mixed Nuts:

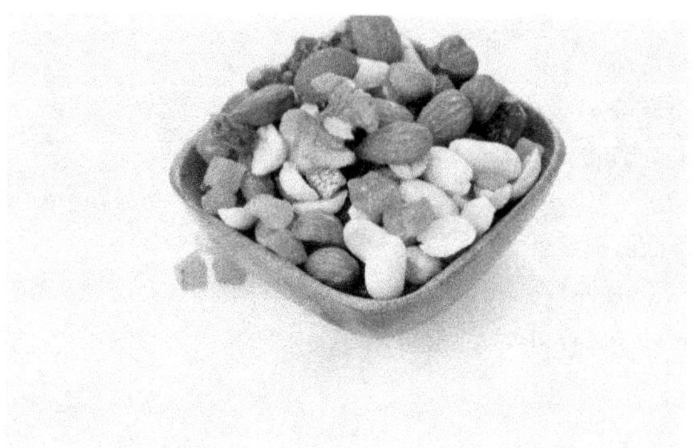

Ingredients:

- 2 cups mixed nuts (almonds, walnuts, cashews, pecans, etc.)
- 1 tablespoon melted butter or olive oil
- 1 tablespoon honey or maple syrup (optional)
- 1 teaspoon salt (adjust to taste)
- 1/2 teaspoon ground cinnamon (optional)
- 1/4 teaspoon cayenne pepper (optional, for a spicy kick)

Instructions:

1. Preheat your oven to 350°F (175°C).
2. In a large bowl, mix the mixed nuts with melted butter or olive oil until evenly coated.
3. If desired, drizzle honey or maple syrup over the nuts for a touch of sweetness.
4. Sprinkle salt evenly over the nuts. Adjust the amount based on your taste preference.
5. Optional: Add ground cinnamon for a warm, aromatic flavor, and cayenne pepper for a spicy element. Toss everything together to coat the nuts evenly.

6. Spread the coated nuts in a single layer on a baking sheet lined with parchment paper.

7. Roast the nuts in the preheated oven for 10-15 minutes, stirring halfway through, until they are golden brown and fragrant.

8. Keep a close eye on them, as nuts can burn quickly.

9. Once roasted, remove the nuts from the oven and let them cool completely.

10. Store the roasted mixed nuts in an airtight container.

Hard-Boiled Eggs:

Ingredients:

- Eggs (as many as you desire)

Instructions:

1. Place the eggs in a single layer in a saucepan or pot. Use eggs that are not too fresh, as slightly older eggs are easier to peel.

2. Add enough water to the pot to cover the eggs by about an inch.

3. Place the pot on the stove over medium-high heat and bring the water to a gentle boil.

4. Once the water is boiling, reduce the heat to low, cover the pot with a lid, and let the eggs simmer for 9-12 minutes.

5. For medium-sized eggs, 9 minutes will give you a slightly soft center, while 12 minutes will yield a fully-cooked hard-boiled egg.

6. While the eggs are cooking, prepare a bowl of ice water.

7. Once the eggs have finished cooking, use a slotted spoon to transfer them immediately to the ice water. Let them sit for at least 5 minutes to cool and stop the cooking process.

8. Gently tap each egg on a hard surface to crack the shell, then roll it between your hands to loosen the shell. Peel the shell starting from the wider end, where the air pocket is usually located.

9. Rinse the peeled eggs under cold water to remove any remaining shell pieces.

10. Your hard-boiled eggs are now ready to be enjoyed as a snack, added to salads, or used in various recipes.

Sliced Turkey:

Ingredients:

- 1 pound turkey breast (cooked and cooled)
- 1 tablespoon olive oil
- 1 teaspoon dried thyme
- 1 teaspoon garlic powder
- 1 teaspoon onion powder
- Salt and black pepper to taste

Instructions:

1. Cook the Turkey:
   - You can use leftover roasted or grilled turkey, or cook the turkey breast specifically for slicing. Season the turkey breast with salt, pepper, and any desired herbs or spices.
   - Roast or grill the turkey breast until it reaches an internal temperature of 165°F (74°C). Let it cool completely.
2. Slice the Turkey:
   - Once the turkey is cooled, use a sharp knife to slice it thinly. The slices can be adjusted based on your preference.
3. Seasoning:
   - In a bowl, mix olive oil, dried thyme, garlic powder, onion powder, salt, and black pepper.
4. Coat the Sliced Turkey:
   - Drizzle the seasoning mixture over the sliced turkey and toss gently to ensure the slices are evenly coated.
5. Serve:

o   Arrange the seasoned sliced turkey on a platter or use it in sandwiches, wraps, salads, or any other dish as desired.

6. Storage:

    o   Store any leftover sliced turkey in an airtight container in the refrigerator for up to 3-4 days.

Greek Yogurt with Berries:

Ingredients:

- 1 cup Greek yogurt (plain or vanilla)
- 1 cup mixed berries (strawberries, blueberries, raspberries)
- 1 tablespoon honey or maple syrup
- 1/4 cup granola (optional, for crunch)
- Fresh mint leaves (optional, for garnish)

Instructions:

1. Prepare the Berries:

    o   Rinse the berries under cold water and pat them dry with a paper towel.

    o   If using strawberries, hull and slice them.

2. Assemble the Bowl:

    o   Spoon Greek yogurt into a serving bowl.

3. Add Berries:

    o   Arrange the mixed berries on top of the Greek yogurt.

4. Drizzle with Sweetener:

    o   Drizzle honey or maple syrup over the yogurt and berries for sweetness. Adjust the amount based on your preference.

5. Optional Crunch:

    o   If desired, sprinkle granola over the top to add a crunchy texture.

6. Garnish (Optional):

    o   Garnish with fresh mint leaves for a burst of freshness.

7. Serve:

- o Serve immediately and enjoy your delicious and nutritious Greek Yogurt with Berries.

Hummus and Veggie Sticks:

Ingredients:

- 1 can (15 oz) chickpeas, drained and rinsed (reserve a few for garnish)
- 1/4 cup tahini
- 2 tablespoons lemon juice
- 2 cloves garlic, minced
- 1/2 teaspoon ground cumin
- 1/4 teaspoon paprika (plus extra for garnish)
- Salt and black pepper to taste
- 2-3 tablespoons olive oil (plus extra for drizzling)
- Carrot sticks, cucumber slices, bell pepper strips, and other veggies for dipping

Instructions:

1. Prepare the Hummus:
   - o In a food processor, combine chickpeas, tahini, lemon juice, minced garlic, ground cumin, paprika, salt, and black pepper.
2. Blend:
   - o Blend the ingredients until smooth. If the mixture is too thick, you can add a tablespoon of water at a time until you reach your desired consistency.
3. Adjust Seasoning:
   - o Taste and adjust the seasoning, adding more salt, pepper, or lemon juice if needed.
4. Drizzle Olive Oil:
   - o While blending, drizzle in the olive oil to create a creamy and smooth texture.
5. Prepare Veggie Sticks:
   - o Wash and cut an assortment of veggies into sticks or slices for dipping.

6. Serve:

   - Transfer the hummus to a serving bowl. Garnish with a drizzle of olive oil, a sprinkle of paprika, and a few whole chickpeas.

Trail Mix:

Ingredients:

- 1 cup nuts (almonds, cashews, walnuts)
- 1 cup seeds (pumpkin seeds, sunflower seeds)
- 1 cup dried fruit (raisins, cranberries, apricots)
- 1 cup whole grain cereal or pretzels
- 1/2 cup dark chocolate chips or chunks
- 1/2 cup coconut flakes (optional)
- 1/2 teaspoon cinnamon (optional)
- 1/4 teaspoon salt

Instructions:

1. Select Ingredients:
   - Choose a variety of nuts, seeds, dried fruit, and other optional ingredients based on your preferences.
2. Preheat Oven (Optional):
   - If desired, preheat your oven to 350°F (175°C).
3. Toast Nuts and Seeds (Optional):
   - Spread nuts and seeds on a baking sheet and toast in the oven for about 8-10 minutes, or until they are golden brown. This step enhances their flavor but is optional.
4. Combine Ingredients:
   - In a large bowl, combine the toasted or untoasted nuts and seeds with dried fruit, whole grain cereal or pretzels, chocolate chips or chunks, coconut flakes (if using), cinnamon (if using), and salt.
5. Mix Well:

- ○ Toss all the ingredients together until they are evenly distributed.

6. Store:

  - ○ Transfer the trail mix to an airtight container for storage.

7. Enjoy:

  - ○ Grab a handful of this homemade trail mix for a quick and satisfying snack. It's perfect for hikes, road trips, or a boost of energy during the day.

Cottage Cheese with Pineapple:

Ingredients:

- 1 cup cottage cheese
- 1 cup fresh pineapple chunks (or canned pineapple tidbits, drained)
- 1 tablespoon honey or maple syrup (optional, for sweetness)
- Fresh mint leaves for garnish (optional)

Instructions:

1. Prepare Cottage Cheese:

  - ○ Scoop 1 cup of cottage cheese into a serving bowl.

2. Add Pineapple:

  - ○ Add 1 cup of fresh pineapple chunks or drained canned pineapple tidbits to the cottage cheese.

3. Sweeten (Optional):

  - ○ If you desire additional sweetness, drizzle honey or maple syrup over the cottage cheese and pineapple. Adjust the amount based on your taste preference.

4. Mix Gently:

  - ○ Gently stir the cottage cheese and pineapple together to combine the flavors.

5. Garnish (Optional):

  - ○ Garnish with fresh mint leaves for a touch of freshness.

6. Serve:

   ○ Serve the cottage cheese with pineapple immediately as a refreshing and protein-packed snack or breakfast option.

Apple with Almond Butter:

Ingredients:

- 2 medium-sized apples (any variety)
- 1/2 cup almond butter
- 1 tablespoon honey (optional)
- 1/4 teaspoon cinnamon
- Sliced almonds for garnish (optional)

Instructions:

1. Wash and core the apples, then cut them into thin slices or wedges.
2. In a microwave-safe bowl or on the stovetop, gently warm the almond butter until it becomes smooth and easily spreadable.
3. Optional: Stir in honey to the almond butter for added sweetness.
4. Arrange the apple slices on a serving plate.
5. Using a knife or spoon, generously spread almond butter over each apple slice.
6. Sprinkle cinnamon over the almond butter-covered apples.
7. Optionally, garnish with sliced almonds for added crunch and visual appeal.
8. Serve immediately and enjoy this delightful and healthy apple with almond butter snack!

Edamame:

Ingredients:

- 2 cups frozen edamame in pods
- 1 tablespoon sea salt
- Optional: Sesame seeds, chili flakes, or soy sauce for seasoning

Instructions:

1. Bring a pot of water to a boil. Add the sea salt.

2. Add the frozen edamame pods to the boiling water.

3. Cook the edamame for 3-5 minutes, or until they are tender.

4. Drain the edamame and transfer them to a bowl.

5. If desired, sprinkle sesame seeds, chili flakes, or drizzle soy sauce over the edamame for added flavor.

6. Toss the edamame gently to coat them evenly with the seasoning.

7. Serve the edamame either warm or at room temperature.

8. To eat, simply squeeze the pods, and the beans will pop out into your mouth. Discard the pods.

Sardines on Whole-Grain Crackers:

Ingredients:

- 1 can (about 4 oz) of sardines in olive oil, drained
- Whole-grain crackers
- 1 tablespoon lemon juice
- 1 tablespoon chopped fresh parsley
- Salt and pepper to taste
- Optional: Dijon mustard for added flavor

Instructions:

1. Open the can of sardines and drain them from the oil.

2. In a bowl, flake the sardines with a fork, breaking them into smaller pieces.

3. Squeeze fresh lemon juice over the flaked sardines and mix well.

4. Season with salt and pepper to taste. If desired, add a dollop of Dijon mustard for extra flavor.

5. Chop fresh parsley and sprinkle it over the sardines.

6. Arrange the whole-grain crackers on a serving plate.

7. Spoon the seasoned sardines onto each cracker.

8. Garnish with additional parsley if desired.

9. Serve immediately and enjoy this quick and nutritious sardines on whole-grain crackers snack!

Avocado and Tomato Slices:

Ingredients:

- 2 ripe avocados
- 2 large tomatoes
- Olive oil
- Balsamic vinegar
- Salt and pepper to taste
- Fresh basil leaves for garnish (optional)

Instructions:

1. Slice the avocados and tomatoes into even, thin slices.
2. Arrange the avocado and tomato slices on a serving plate, alternating them for a visually appealing presentation.
3. Drizzle olive oil and balsamic vinegar over the avocado and tomato slices.
4. Season with salt and pepper to taste.
5. Optional: Garnish with fresh basil leaves for added flavor and aroma.
6. Allow the dish to marinate for a few minutes to let the flavors meld.
7. Serve immediately and enjoy this simple, refreshing, and healthy avocado and tomato slices dish as a snack or a light appetizer!

Popcorn:

Ingredients:

- 1/2 cup popcorn kernels
- 3 tablespoons vegetable oil or coconut oil
- Salt to taste
- Optional: Butter for drizzling

Instructions:

1. Place a large, heavy-bottomed pot with a lid on the stove over medium heat.

2. Add the vegetable oil or coconut oil to the pot.

3. Drop a few popcorn kernels into the oil. Once they pop, the oil is hot enough.

4. Add the remaining popcorn kernels to the pot and cover it with the lid.

5. Shake the pot gently to ensure the kernels are evenly coated with oil.

6. Allow the popcorn to pop, shaking the pot occasionally to prevent burning.

7. Once the popping slows down (usually after 2-3 seconds between pops), remove the pot from the heat.

8. Carefully open the lid, keeping it away from your face to avoid steam.

9. Season the popcorn with salt to taste, and drizzle with melted butter if desired. Toss to coat evenly.

10. Transfer the popcorn to a large bowl and enjoy your homemade popcorn for a movie night or snack time!

(Satisfying Appetizers)

Stuffed Mushrooms:

Ingredients:

- 20 large white or cremini mushrooms, cleaned and stems removed
- 1/2 cup cream cheese, softened
- 1/4 cup grated Parmesan cheese
- 2 cloves garlic, minced
- 2 tablespoons chopped fresh parsley
- Salt and pepper to taste
- Olive oil for brushing

Instructions:

1. Preheat the oven to 375°F (190°C).

2. Place the cleaned mushroom caps on a baking sheet, cap side down.

3. In a bowl, mix together cream cheese, grated Parmesan, minced garlic, chopped parsley, salt, and pepper until well combined.

4. Spoon the cream cheese mixture into each mushroom cap, pressing it down gently.

5. Brush the mushroom caps with olive oil for a golden finish.

6. Bake in the preheated oven for 15-20 minutes or until the mushrooms are tender and the filling is golden brown.

7. Remove from the oven and let them cool slightly before serving.

8. Garnish with additional chopped parsley if desired.

9. Serve these delicious stuffed mushrooms as an appetizer or party snack!

Shrimp Cocktail:

Ingredients:

For the Shrimp:

- 1 pound large shrimp, peeled and deveined
- 1 tablespoon olive oil
- Salt and pepper to taste
- Lemon wedges for serving

For the Cocktail Sauce:

- 1/2 cup ketchup
- 2 tablespoons horseradish (adjust to taste)
- 1 tablespoon lemon juice
- 1 teaspoon Worcestershire sauce
- Dash of hot sauce (optional)
- Salt and pepper to taste

Instructions:

1. Preheat the oven to 400°F (200°C).

2. Toss the peeled and deveined shrimp with olive oil, salt, and pepper.

3. Place the seasoned shrimp on a baking sheet and bake for 8-10 minutes or until they are pink and opaque.

4. While the shrimp are baking, prepare the cocktail sauce. In a bowl, combine ketchup, horseradish, lemon juice, Worcestershire sauce, hot sauce (if using), salt, and pepper. Adjust horseradish and hot sauce to your taste preference.

5. Once the shrimp are cooked, let them cool for a few minutes.

6. Arrange the shrimp on a serving platter with lemon wedges.

7. Serve the shrimp with the cocktail sauce on the side for dipping.

Vegetable Crudité with Tzatziki:

Ingredients:

For the Tzatziki:

- 1 cup Greek yogurt
- 1 cucumber, finely diced
- 2 cloves garlic, minced
- 1 tablespoon fresh dill, chopped
- 1 tablespoon lemon juice
- Salt and pepper to taste

For the Vegetable Crudité:

- Assorted fresh vegetables (carrots, cucumbers, bell peppers, cherry tomatoes, etc.), washed and sliced

Instructions:

Tzatziki:

1. In a bowl, combine Greek yogurt, finely diced cucumber, minced garlic, chopped dill, and lemon juice.

2. Mix well until all ingredients are evenly incorporated.

3. Season the tzatziki with salt and pepper to taste. Refrigerate for at least 30 minutes to allow the flavors to meld.

Vegetable Crudité:

1. Wash and prepare a variety of fresh vegetables by slicing them into sticks or bite-sized pieces.

2. Arrange the vegetable slices on a serving platter.

3. Take the tzatziki out of the refrigerator and give it a final stir.

4. Place the bowl of tzatziki in the center of the vegetable platter or serve it in a separate bowl for dipping.

5. Serve the vegetable crudité with tzatziki as a refreshing and healthy appetizer.

6. Enjoy the crisp vegetables paired with the cool and tangy tzatziki dip!

Smoked Salmon Roll-Ups:

Ingredients:

- 8 slices smoked salmon
- 1/2 cup cream cheese, softened
- 1 tablespoon capers, drained
- 1 tablespoon red onion, finely chopped
- 1 tablespoon fresh dill, chopped
- Zest of one lemon
- Freshly ground black pepper
- 1 cucumber, thinly sliced (optional, for wrapping)

Instructions:

1. In a bowl, mix together the softened cream cheese, capers, chopped red onion, fresh dill, lemon zest, and a pinch of freshly ground black pepper.

2. Lay out the smoked salmon slices on a clean surface.

3. Spread a thin layer of the cream cheese mixture evenly over each slice of smoked salmon.

4. If using cucumber, place a thin slice along the edge of each salmon slice.

5. Starting from one end, carefully roll up each slice into a tight roll.

6. Optional: Secure the rolls with toothpicks and refrigerate for 15-20 minutes to firm up.

7. Once chilled, slice the rolls into bite-sized pieces.

8. Arrange the smoked salmon roll-ups on a serving plate and garnish with additional dill or lemon zest if desired.

9. Serve as an elegant appetizer or light snack.

Guacamole with Jicama Sticks:

Ingredients:

For the Guacamole:

- 3 ripe avocados
- 1 small red onion, finely diced
- 1-2 tomatoes, diced
- 1 jalapeño, seeded and finely chopped (optional)
- 1/4 cup fresh cilantro, chopped
- 2 cloves garlic, minced
- Juice of 1-2 limes
- Salt and pepper to taste

For the Jicama Sticks:

- 1 medium jicama, peeled and cut into thin sticks

Instructions:

Guacamole:

1. Cut the avocados in half, remove the pits, and scoop the flesh into a bowl.
2. Mash the avocados with a fork or potato masher until smooth or slightly chunky, depending on your preference.
3. Add the finely diced red onion, diced tomatoes, chopped jalapeño (if using), minced garlic, and chopped cilantro to the mashed avocados.
4. Squeeze lime juice over the mixture and season with salt and pepper to taste.
5. Mix all the ingredients together until well combined.

Jicama Sticks:

1. Peel the jicama and cut it into thin sticks resembling french fries.
2. Arrange the jicama sticks on a serving platter.

Serving:

1. Serve the guacamole in a bowl, surrounded by the jicama sticks.

2. Use the jicama sticks to scoop up the delicious guacamole and enjoy this refreshing and crunchy snack.

3. Optionally, garnish the guacamole with additional cilantro or a sprinkle of paprika.

4. Enjoy your Guacamole with Jicama Sticks as a healthy and flavorful appetizer or snack!

Quinoa Salad Cups:

Ingredients:

For the Quinoa Salad:

- 1 cup quinoa, rinsed and cooked according to package instructions
- 1 cup cherry tomatoes, halved
- 1 cucumber, diced
- 1 bell pepper (any color), diced
- 1/4 cup red onion, finely chopped
- 1/4 cup feta cheese, crumbled
- 1/4 cup Kalamata olives, sliced
- 2 tablespoons fresh parsley, chopped

For the Lemon Vinaigrette:

- 3 tablespoons extra-virgin olive oil
- Juice of 1 lemon
- 1 teaspoon Dijon mustard
- 1 clove garlic, minced
- Salt and pepper to taste

For Assembling:

- Small lettuce leaves or endive cups

Instructions:

Quinoa Salad:

1. Cook the quinoa according to package instructions and let it cool.
2. In a large bowl, combine the cooked quinoa, cherry tomatoes, diced cucumber, diced bell pepper, finely chopped red onion, crumbled feta cheese, sliced Kalamata olives, and chopped fresh parsley.

Lemon Vinaigrette:

1. In a small bowl, whisk together the extra-virgin olive oil, lemon juice, Dijon mustard, minced garlic, salt, and pepper.
2. Pour the vinaigrette over the quinoa salad and toss until everything is well coated.

Assembling:

1. Spoon the quinoa salad into small lettuce leaves or endive cups, creating bite-sized cups.
2. Arrange the quinoa salad cups on a serving platter.
3. Optionally, garnish with extra feta cheese and parsley.
4. Serve immediately and enjoy these refreshing and nutritious quinoa salad cups as a light appetizer or party snack!

Stuffed Bell Peppers:

Ingredients:

- 4 large bell peppers, halved and seeds removed
- 1 pound ground beef or turkey
- 1 cup cooked quinoa or rice
- 1 cup black beans, drained and rinsed
- 1 cup corn kernels (fresh, frozen, or canned)
- 1 cup diced tomatoes
- 1 cup shredded cheese (cheddar, Monterey Jack, or your choice)
- 1/2 cup diced red onion
- 2 cloves garlic, minced
- 1 teaspoon chili powder
- 1 teaspoon cumin
- Salt and pepper to taste
- Olive oil for drizzling
- Fresh cilantro or parsley for garnish (optional)

Instructions:

1. Preheat the oven to 375°F (190°C).
2. Place the halved bell peppers in a baking dish, cut side up.
3. In a large skillet, cook the ground beef or turkey over medium heat until browned. Drain any excess fat.
4. Add minced garlic and diced red onion to the skillet, sautéing until softened.
5. Stir in the cooked quinoa or rice, black beans, corn, diced tomatoes, chili powder, cumin, salt, and pepper. Cook for an additional 2-3 minutes.
6. Remove the skillet from heat and let the mixture cool slightly.

7. Stuff each bell pepper half with the meat and vegetable mixture, pressing it down gently.
8. Drizzle a bit of olive oil over the stuffed bell peppers.
9. Sprinkle shredded cheese on top of each stuffed pepper.
10. Cover the baking dish with aluminum foil and bake in the preheated oven for 25-30 minutes or until the peppers are tender.
11. If desired, broil for an additional 2-3 minutes to melt and slightly brown the cheese.
12. Garnish with fresh cilantro or parsley.
13. Serve the stuffed bell peppers hot, and enjoy this wholesome and flavorful meal!

Olive Tapenade:

Ingredients:

- 1 cup pitted Kalamata olives
- 1/2 cup green olives
- 2 cloves garlic, minced
- 2 tablespoons capers, drained
- 2 tablespoons fresh parsley, chopped
- 1 tablespoon fresh lemon juice
- 1/4 cup extra-virgin olive oil
- Freshly ground black pepper, to taste

Instructions:

1. In a food processor, combine the Kalamata olives, green olives, minced garlic, capers, and fresh parsley.
2. Pulse the ingredients until coarsely chopped, scraping down the sides of the bowl as needed.
3. Add the fresh lemon juice to the olive mixture and pulse a few more times.
4. With the food processor running, gradually stream in the extra-virgin olive oil until the tapenade reaches your desired consistency.

5. Taste and season with freshly ground black pepper as needed; additional salt is usually unnecessary due to the saltiness of the olives and capers.

6. Transfer the olive tapenade to a bowl.

7. Cover and refrigerate for at least 30 minutes to allow the flavors to meld.

8. Before serving, bring the tapenade to room temperature and give it a stir.

9. Serve the olive tapenade with crusty bread, crackers, or as a flavorful accompaniment to various dishes.

Ceviche:

Ingredients:

- 1 pound fresh white fish (tilapia, sea bass, or snapper), cut into small cubes
- 1 cup fresh lime juice (about 8-10 limes)
- 1 red onion, thinly sliced
- 1-2 tomatoes, diced
- 1 cucumber, peeled and diced
- 1 jalapeño, seeded and finely chopped
- 1/2 cup fresh cilantro, chopped
- Salt and pepper to taste
- Avocado slices for garnish (optional)
- Corn tortilla chips for serving

Instructions:

1. In a non-reactive bowl (glass or ceramic), place the fish cubes and cover them with fresh lime juice. Make sure the fish is fully submerged. Allow it to marinate for at least 30 minutes to 1 hour, or until the fish turns opaque and "cooked" in the lime juice.

2. Drain the lime juice from the fish, reserving a small amount for later.

3. Add the thinly sliced red onion, diced tomatoes, diced cucumber, chopped jalapeño, and chopped cilantro to the fish.

4. Gently toss the ingredients together, ensuring an even distribution.

5. Season the ceviche with salt and pepper to taste. If needed, add a bit of the reserved lime juice for extra acidity.

6. Cover the bowl with plastic wrap and refrigerate for at least 30 minutes to allow the flavors to meld.

7. Before serving, give the ceviche a final toss.

8. Garnish with avocado slices if desired.

9. Serve the ceviche chilled, either in a bowl or individual cups, accompanied by corn tortilla chips.

Grilled Asparagus:

Ingredients:

- 1 bunch fresh asparagus spears
- 2 tablespoons olive oil
- 2 cloves garlic, minced
- Salt and black pepper to taste
- Lemon wedges for serving

Instructions:

1. Preheat the grill to medium-high heat.

2. Wash and trim the tough ends off the asparagus spears.

3. In a small bowl, mix together olive oil and minced garlic.

4. Drizzle the olive oil and garlic mixture over the asparagus spears, ensuring they are evenly coated.

5. Season the asparagus with salt and black pepper to taste.

6. Place the asparagus spears on the preheated grill, arranging them perpendicular to the grates to prevent them from falling through.

7. Grill the asparagus for about 5-7 minutes, turning occasionally, or until they are tender and have slight char marks.

8. Remove the grilled asparagus from the heat.

9. Squeeze fresh lemon juice over the grilled asparagus before serving.

10. Serve immediately as a delicious side dish or appetizer.

Caprese Skewers:

Ingredients:

- Cherry tomatoes
- Fresh mozzarella balls (bocconcini)
- Fresh basil leaves
- Balsamic glaze
- Extra-virgin olive oil
- Salt and black pepper to taste
- Wooden skewers

Instructions:

1. Prepare the wooden skewers by soaking them in water for about 30 minutes to prevent them from burning during grilling.
2. Rinse the cherry tomatoes and pat them dry.
3. Thread a cherry tomato onto the skewer, followed by a fresh basil leaf, and then a mozzarella ball.
4. Repeat the pattern until the skewer is filled, leaving a bit of space at the ends for easy handling.
5. Arrange the Caprese skewers on a serving platter.
6. Drizzle extra-virgin olive oil and balsamic glaze over the skewers.
7. Sprinkle salt and black pepper to taste.
8. Optionally, garnish with additional fresh basil leaves for presentation.
9. Serve the Caprese skewers as a delightful and refreshing appetizer.

Sushi Rolls:

Ingredients:

For the Sushi Rice:

- 2 cups sushi rice

- 2 1/2 cups water
- 1/3 cup rice vinegar
- 3 tablespoons sugar
- 1 teaspoon salt

For the Sushi Rolls:

- Nori (seaweed) sheets
- Fresh fish (like tuna or salmon), thinly sliced
- Vegetables (avocado, cucumber, carrot), julienned
- Soy sauce for dipping
- Pickled ginger and wasabi for serving

Instructions:

Sushi Rice:

1. Rinse the sushi rice under cold water until the water runs clear.
2. Combine the rice and water in a rice cooker and cook according to the manufacturer's instructions.
3. While the rice is still hot, transfer it to a large bowl and gently fold in a mixture of rice vinegar, sugar, and salt. Allow the rice to cool to room temperature.

Sushi Rolls:

1. Place a bamboo sushi rolling mat on a flat surface and put a sheet of plastic wrap on top. Lay a sheet of nori, shiny side down, on the plastic wrap.
2. Wet your hands to prevent the rice from sticking, and spread a thin layer of sushi rice over the nori, leaving about 1 inch at the top.
3. Arrange thin slices of fish and julienned vegetables in the center of the rice.
4. Starting from the edge closest to you, lift the bamboo mat with the plastic wrap and rice, rolling it over the filling. Apply gentle pressure to shape the roll.
5. Moisten the top edge of the nori with a little water to seal the roll.
6. Use a sharp knife to slice the roll into bite-sized pieces.
7. Repeat the process with different combinations of fish and vegetables for variety.
8. Serve the sushi rolls with soy sauce, pickled ginger, and wasabi.

CHAPTER 6: SOUPS AND STEW

Lentil Soup:

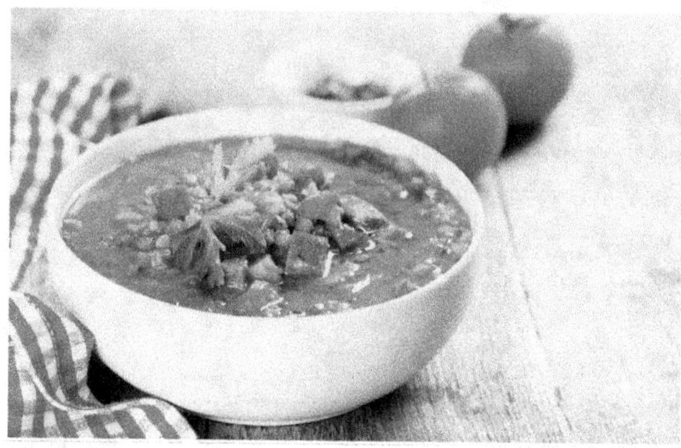

Ingredients:

- 1 cup dry green or brown lentils, rinsed and drained
- 1 onion, finely chopped
- 2 carrots, peeled and diced
- 2 celery stalks, diced
- 3 cloves garlic, minced
- 1 can (14 oz) diced tomatoes
- 6 cups vegetable or chicken broth
- 1 teaspoon ground cumin
- 1 teaspoon ground coriander
- 1 teaspoon smoked paprika
- 1 bay leaf
- Salt and pepper to taste
- 2 tablespoons olive oil
- Fresh parsley for garnish (optional)

- Lemon wedges for serving (optional)

Instructions:

1. In a large pot, heat the olive oil over medium heat. Add chopped onion, carrots, and celery. Cook until vegetables are softened, about 5-7 minutes.
2. Add minced garlic, ground cumin, ground coriander, and smoked paprika. Stir and cook for an additional 2 minutes until fragrant.
3. Add the rinsed lentils, diced tomatoes (with their juice), bay leaf, and broth to the pot. Stir well.
4. Bring the soup to a boil, then reduce the heat to low, cover, and simmer for about 25-30 minutes or until the lentils are tender.
5. Season the lentil soup with salt and pepper to taste. Adjust the seasoning if needed.
6. Remove the bay leaf before serving.
7. Ladle the soup into bowls and garnish with fresh parsley if desired.
8. Serve the lentil soup hot, optionally with lemon wedges on the side for a burst of citrus flavor.

Miso Soup:

Ingredients:

- 4 cups dashi (Japanese soup stock) or vegetable broth
- 3 tablespoons white or light yellow miso paste
- 1 cup firm tofu, diced
- 2 green onions, thinly sliced
- 1 cup fresh mushrooms, sliced (shiitake or enoki mushrooms work well)
- 1 cup seaweed (wakame), rehydrated and chopped
- 1 tablespoon soy sauce (optional)
- 1 teaspoon sesame oil (optional)
- Fresh cilantro or sliced radishes for garnish (optional)

Instructions:

1. In a pot, bring the dashi or vegetable broth to a simmer over medium heat.

2. While the broth is heating, rehydrate the seaweed (wakame) according to the package instructions.

3. Once the broth is simmering, add the diced tofu, sliced green onions, and mushrooms. Simmer for about 5 minutes until the vegetables are tender.

4. In a small bowl, whisk together the miso paste with a ladleful of hot broth until the miso is fully dissolved.

5. Lower the heat, add the dissolved miso paste to the pot, and stir well.

6. If desired, add soy sauce and sesame oil for extra flavor. Adjust the seasoning according to taste.

7. Add the rehydrated and chopped seaweed to the pot, stirring gently.

8. Simmer the miso soup for an additional 2-3 minutes without boiling to preserve the miso's beneficial enzymes.

9. Remove the pot from heat and let it sit for a minute.

10. Ladle the miso soup into bowls, garnish with fresh cilantro or sliced radishes if desired.

11. Serve the miso soup hot as a comforting and flavorful appetizer or light meal.

Chicken and Vegetable Soup:

Ingredients:

- 1 pound boneless, skinless chicken breasts or thighs, diced
- 1 tablespoon olive oil
- 1 onion, finely chopped
- 2 carrots, peeled and sliced
- 2 celery stalks, sliced
- 3 cloves garlic, minced
- 8 cups chicken broth
- 1 cup diced tomatoes (fresh or canned)
- 1 cup green beans, chopped
- 1 cup corn kernels (fresh, frozen, or canned)

- 1 cup peas (fresh or frozen)
- 1 teaspoon dried thyme
- 1 teaspoon dried rosemary
- Salt and pepper to taste
- 1 cup pasta or rice (optional)
- Fresh parsley for garnish (optional)

Instructions:

1. In a large pot, heat olive oil over medium heat. Add diced chicken and cook until browned. Remove the chicken from the pot and set it aside.
2. In the same pot, add chopped onion, sliced carrots, sliced celery, and minced garlic. Cook until the vegetables are softened, about 5-7 minutes.
3. Pour in the chicken broth, diced tomatoes, green beans, corn, and peas. Add the dried thyme and rosemary. Bring the soup to a boil.
4. If using pasta or rice, add it to the pot and cook according to the package instructions.
5. Reduce the heat to a simmer, add the cooked chicken back to the pot, and let the soup simmer for an additional 10-15 minutes.
6. Season the soup with salt and pepper to taste.
7. Ladle the chicken and vegetable soup into bowls.
8. Garnish with fresh parsley if desired.
9. Serve the soup hot, and enjoy a comforting and nutritious meal!

Tomato Basil Soup:

Ingredients:

- 2 tablespoons olive oil
- 1 onion, chopped
- 3 cloves garlic, minced
- 2 cans (28 oz each) whole peeled tomatoes
- 1 can (14 oz) crushed tomatoes

- 4 cups vegetable or chicken broth
- 1/2 cup fresh basil leaves, chopped
- 1 teaspoon dried oregano
- 1 teaspoon sugar (optional, to balance acidity)
- Salt and black pepper to taste
- 1/2 cup heavy cream (optional, for creamier soup)
- Grated Parmesan cheese for garnish (optional)
- Croutons or bread for serving

Instructions:

1. In a large pot, heat olive oil over medium heat. Add chopped onion and sauté until softened, about 5 minutes.
2. Add minced garlic and sauté for an additional 1-2 minutes until fragrant.
3. Pour in the whole peeled tomatoes, crushed tomatoes, and broth. Break up the whole tomatoes using a spoon.
4. Add chopped basil, dried oregano, and sugar (if using). Stir well.
5. Season the soup with salt and black pepper to taste. Bring the mixture to a simmer.
6. Reduce the heat to low and let the soup simmer for about 20-25 minutes to allow the flavors to meld.
7. Use an immersion blender to blend the soup until smooth. Alternatively, transfer the soup in batches to a blender.
8. If using heavy cream, stir it into the soup to add creaminess. Adjust the seasoning if needed.
9. Ladle the tomato basil soup into bowls.
10. Garnish with grated Parmesan cheese and additional fresh basil if desired.
11. Serve the soup hot with croutons or a side of crusty bread.

Spicy Black Bean Soup:

Ingredients:

- 2 cans (15 oz each) black beans, drained and rinsed

- 1 tablespoon olive oil
- 1 onion, chopped
- 3 cloves garlic, minced
- 1 jalapeño, seeded and finely chopped
- 1 red bell pepper, diced
- 1 carrot, peeled and diced
- 1 teaspoon ground cumin
- 1 teaspoon chili powder
- 1/2 teaspoon smoked paprika
- 4 cups vegetable or chicken broth
- 1 can (14 oz) diced tomatoes
- Salt and black pepper to taste
- Juice of 1 lime
- Fresh cilantro for garnish
- Sour cream or Greek yogurt for serving (optional)

Instructions:

1. In a large pot, heat olive oil over medium heat. Add chopped onion, minced garlic, jalapeño, diced red bell pepper, and diced carrot. Sauté until the vegetables are softened, about 5-7 minutes.
2. Add ground cumin, chili powder, and smoked paprika. Stir well to coat the vegetables in the spices.
3. Pour in the black beans, vegetable or chicken broth, and diced tomatoes (with their juice). Bring the soup to a boil.
4. Reduce the heat to low and let the soup simmer for about 15-20 minutes to allow the flavors to meld.
5. Season the soup with salt and black pepper to taste.
6. Use an immersion blender to partially blend the soup, leaving some whole beans for texture. Alternatively, transfer a portion of the soup to a blender and blend before returning it to the pot.

7. Stir in the lime juice for a burst of freshness.

8. Ladle the spicy black bean soup into bowls.

9. Garnish with fresh cilantro and, if desired, a dollop of sour cream or Greek yogurt.

10. Serve the soup hot, and enjoy the hearty and spicy goodness!

Gazpacho:

Ingredients:

- 6 ripe tomatoes, cored and chopped
- 1 cucumber, peeled and chopped
- 1 bell pepper (red or green), chopped
- 1 small red onion, chopped
- 2 cloves garlic, minced
- 4 cups tomato juice
- 1/4 cup red wine vinegar
- 1/4 cup olive oil
- 1 teaspoon sugar
- Salt and black pepper to taste
- 1 teaspoon ground cumin
- 1/2 teaspoon smoked paprika
- Dash of hot sauce (optional)
- Fresh basil or cilantro for garnish
- Croutons for serving (optional)

Instructions:

1. In a blender or food processor, combine chopped tomatoes, cucumber, bell pepper, red onion, and minced garlic.

2. Blend the vegetables until smooth or slightly chunky, depending on your preference.

3. Transfer the blended mixture to a large bowl.

4. Stir in tomato juice, red wine vinegar, olive oil, sugar, salt, black pepper, ground cumin, smoked paprika, and hot sauce (if using). Mix well.

5. Taste the gazpacho and adjust the seasoning if needed.

6. Cover the bowl and refrigerate the gazpacho for at least 2 hours, allowing the flavors to meld and the soup to chill.

7. Before serving, stir the gazpacho and check the consistency. If it's too thick, you can add more tomato juice.

8. Ladle the chilled gazpacho into bowls.

9. Garnish with fresh basil or cilantro.

10. Optionally, serve with croutons for added texture.

11. Enjoy this refreshing and vibrant cold soup as a light appetizer or summer meal!

Cream of Mushroom Soup:

Ingredients:

- 1/4 cup unsalted butter
- 1 onion, finely chopped
- 2 cloves garlic, minced
- 1 pound mushrooms, cleaned and sliced
- 1/4 cup all-purpose flour
- 4 cups vegetable or chicken broth
- 1 cup heavy cream
- Salt and black pepper to taste
- 1/2 teaspoon dried thyme
- 1 bay leaf
- Chopped fresh parsley for garnish

Instructions:

1. In a large pot, melt the butter over medium heat.

2. Add finely chopped onion and sauté until softened, about 5 minutes.

3. Stir in minced garlic and sliced mushrooms. Cook until the mushrooms release their moisture and become golden brown.

4. Sprinkle all-purpose flour over the mushroom mixture and stir well to coat.

5. Gradually pour in the vegetable or chicken broth, stirring constantly to avoid lumps. Bring the mixture to a simmer.

6. Add heavy cream, dried thyme, and the bay leaf. Stir well.

7. Simmer the soup for about 15-20 minutes, allowing it to thicken.

8. Season the cream of mushroom soup with salt and black pepper to taste. Adjust the seasoning as needed.

9. Remove the bay leaf from the soup.

10. Using an immersion blender, partially blend the soup to achieve a creamy consistency while leaving some mushroom pieces intact. Alternatively, transfer a portion of the soup to a blender and blend before returning it to the pot.

11. Simmer the soup for an additional 5 minutes to heat through.

12. Ladle the cream of mushroom soup into bowls.

13. Garnish with chopped fresh parsley.

14. Serve the soup hot, and enjoy the rich and comforting flavors

Sweet Potato and Ginger Soup:

Ingredients:

- 2 tablespoons olive oil
- 1 onion, chopped
- 2 cloves garlic, minced
- 1 tablespoon fresh ginger, grated
- 3 large sweet potatoes, peeled and diced
- 4 cups vegetable or chicken broth
- 1 teaspoon ground cumin
- 1/2 teaspoon ground coriander
- 1/2 teaspoon cinnamon

- Pinch of nutmeg
- Salt and black pepper to taste
- 1 can (14 oz) coconut milk
- Juice of 1 orange
- Fresh cilantro for garnish (optional)

Instructions:

1. In a large pot, heat olive oil over medium heat. Add chopped onion and sauté until softened, about 5 minutes.
2. Stir in minced garlic and grated ginger. Cook for an additional 1-2 minutes until fragrant.
3. Add diced sweet potatoes to the pot, along with ground cumin, ground coriander, cinnamon, nutmeg, salt, and black pepper. Stir well to coat the sweet potatoes in the spices.
4. Pour in the vegetable or chicken broth, ensuring the sweet potatoes are fully covered. Bring the mixture to a simmer.
5. Simmer the soup for about 15-20 minutes or until the sweet potatoes are tender.
6. Using an immersion blender, blend the soup until smooth.
7. Stir in coconut milk and orange juice. Continue simmering for an additional 5 minutes.
8. Taste the soup and adjust the seasoning if needed.
9. Ladle the sweet potato and ginger soup into bowls.
10. Optionally, garnish with fresh cilantro.
11. Serve the soup hot, and enjoy the warming and flavorful combination of sweet potatoes and ginger!

Minestrone Soup:

Ingredients:

- 2 tablespoons olive oil
- 1 onion, finely chopped

- 2 carrots, diced
- 2 celery stalks, diced
- 3 cloves garlic, minced
- 1 zucchini, diced
- 1 yellow squash, diced
- 1 cup green beans, cut into bite-sized pieces
- 1 can (14 oz) diced tomatoes
- 1 can (15 oz) cannellini beans, drained and rinsed
- 1/2 cup small pasta (such as ditalini or elbow)
- 6 cups vegetable or chicken broth
- 1 teaspoon dried oregano
- 1 teaspoon dried basil
- 1/2 teaspoon dried thyme
- Salt and black pepper to taste
- 2 cups spinach or kale, chopped
- Grated Parmesan cheese for serving
- Fresh basil for garnish (optional)

Instructions:

1. In a large pot, heat olive oil over medium heat. Add chopped onion, diced carrots, and diced celery. Sauté until the vegetables are softened, about 5-7 minutes.
2. Stir in minced garlic and cook for an additional 1-2 minutes until fragrant.
3. Add diced zucchini, diced yellow squash, green beans, diced tomatoes (with their juice), and drained cannellini beans to the pot. Mix well.
4. Pour in vegetable or chicken broth, and add dried oregano, dried basil, dried thyme, salt, and black pepper. Bring the soup to a boil.
5. Add the small pasta to the pot and simmer until the pasta is al dente.
6. Stir in chopped spinach or kale and cook until wilted.
7. Taste the soup and adjust the seasoning if needed.
8. Ladle the minestrone soup into bowls.

9. Garnish with grated Parmesan cheese and fresh basil if desired.

10. Serve the soup hot and enjoy this hearty and flavorful Italian classic!

Tofu and Spinach Soup:

Ingredients:

- 1 tablespoon sesame oil
- 1 onion, finely chopped
- 2 cloves garlic, minced
- 1-inch piece of ginger, grated
- 4 cups vegetable broth
- 1 block (14 oz) firm tofu, cubed
- 4 cups fresh spinach, chopped
- 2 tablespoons soy sauce
- 1 tablespoon rice vinegar
- 1 teaspoon sugar
- Salt and black pepper to taste
- Green onions for garnish
- Red pepper flakes for optional heat
- Cooked rice or rice noodles (optional, for serving)

Instructions:

1. In a large pot, heat sesame oil over medium heat. Add chopped onion and sauté until softened, about 5 minutes.

2. Stir in minced garlic and grated ginger. Cook for an additional 1-2 minutes until fragrant.

3. Pour in vegetable broth and bring it to a simmer.

4. Add cubed tofu to the pot and simmer for about 5-7 minutes.

5. Stir in chopped spinach and cook until wilted.

6. In a small bowl, mix soy sauce, rice vinegar, sugar, salt, and black pepper. Add this mixture to the soup and stir well.

7. Taste the soup and adjust the seasoning if needed.

8. If desired, add red pepper flakes for a bit of heat.

9. Ladle the tofu and spinach soup into bowls.

10. Garnish with chopped green onions.

11. Optionally, serve the soup over cooked rice or rice noodles.

12. Enjoy this healthy and flavorful Tofu and Spinach Soup as a comforting meal!

Asparagus Soup:

Ingredients:

- 1 bunch fresh asparagus, tough ends trimmed
- 2 tablespoons olive oil
- 1 onion, chopped
- 2 cloves garlic, minced
- 4 cups vegetable or chicken broth
- 1 medium potato, peeled and diced
- 1/2 cup heavy cream (optional, for creamier soup)
- Salt and black pepper to taste
- Fresh lemon juice (from 1 lemon)
- Chopped fresh chives or parsley for garnish

Instructions:

1. Cut the asparagus into 1-inch pieces, reserving a few tips for garnish.

2. In a large pot, heat olive oil over medium heat. Add chopped onion and sauté until softened, about 5 minutes.

3. Add minced garlic and sauté for an additional 1-2 minutes until fragrant.

4. Add asparagus pieces to the pot and cook for about 3-4 minutes.

5. Pour in vegetable or chicken broth, add diced potato, and bring the mixture to a simmer. Cook until the potatoes and asparagus are tender.

6. Using an immersion blender, blend the soup until smooth. Alternatively, transfer a portion of the soup to a blender and blend before returning it to the pot.

7. If using, stir in heavy cream for a creamier texture.

8. Season the soup with salt and black pepper to taste.

9. Squeeze fresh lemon juice into the soup, adjusting to your taste preference.

10. In a small pan, sauté the reserved asparagus tips in a bit of olive oil until they are tender-crisp.

11. Ladle the asparagus soup into bowls.

12. Garnish with sautéed asparagus tips and chopped fresh chives or parsley.

Turkey Chili:

Ingredients:

- 1 tablespoon olive oil
- 1 onion, chopped
- 3 cloves garlic, minced
- 1 pound ground turkey
- 1 bell pepper, diced
- 1 zucchini, diced
- 1 can (14 oz) diced tomatoes
- 1 can (15 oz) kidney beans, drained and rinsed
- 1 can (15 oz) black beans, drained and rinsed
- 2 cups tomato sauce
- 1 cup corn kernels (fresh, frozen, or canned)
- 2 tablespoons chili powder
- 1 teaspoon ground cumin
- 1 teaspoon paprika
- 1/2 teaspoon cayenne pepper (adjust to taste)
- Salt and black pepper to taste
- 2 cups chicken or vegetable broth
- Optional toppings: shredded cheese, sour cream, chopped green onions, cilantro

Instructions:

1. In a large pot, heat olive oil over medium heat. Add chopped onion and sauté until softened, about 5 minutes.
2. Stir in minced garlic and cook for an additional 1-2 minutes until fragrant.
3. Add ground turkey to the pot and cook until browned.
4. Add diced bell pepper and zucchini. Cook for about 3-5 minutes until the vegetables are slightly softened.
5. Pour in diced tomatoes, kidney beans, black beans, tomato sauce, and corn kernels. Stir well.
6. Add chili powder, ground cumin, paprika, cayenne pepper, salt, and black pepper. Mix to combine.
7. Pour in chicken or vegetable broth to achieve your desired consistency.
8. Bring the chili to a simmer and let it cook for at least 20-30 minutes to allow the flavors to meld.
9. Taste and adjust the seasoning as needed.
10. Serve the turkey chili hot, topped with shredded cheese, sour cream, chopped green onions, or cilantro if desired.

Stews:

Beef Stew:

Ingredients:

- 2 pounds beef stew meat, cut into bite-sized cubes
- 2 tablespoons vegetable oil
- 1 onion, chopped
- 3 cloves garlic, minced
- 4 cups beef broth
- 1 cup red wine (optional)
- 2 tablespoons tomato paste
- 1 teaspoon Worcestershire sauce

- 1 bay leaf
- 1 teaspoon dried thyme
- 1 teaspoon dried rosemary
- 4 carrots, peeled and sliced
- 4 potatoes, peeled and diced
- 1 cup frozen peas
- Salt and black pepper to taste
- Chopped fresh parsley for garnish

Instructions:

1. In a large pot or Dutch oven, heat vegetable oil over medium-high heat. Add the beef stew meat and brown on all sides. Remove the beef and set it aside.
2. In the same pot, add chopped onion and sauté until softened, about 5 minutes. Add minced garlic and cook for an additional 1-2 minutes.
3. Pour in beef broth and red wine (if using), scraping the bottom of the pot to release any flavorful bits.
4. Stir in tomato paste, Worcestershire sauce, bay leaf, dried thyme, and dried rosemary.
5. Return the browned beef to the pot and bring the mixture to a simmer. Cover and let it simmer for about 1.5 to 2 hours, or until the meat becomes tender.
6. Add sliced carrots, diced potatoes, and frozen peas to the pot. Season with salt and black pepper to taste.
7. Continue to simmer the stew for an additional 30-45 minutes, or until the vegetables are tender.
8. Taste and adjust the seasoning if needed.
9. Discard the bay leaf.
10. Ladle the beef stew into bowls.
11. Garnish with chopped fresh parsley.
12. Serve the beef stew hot, and enjoy this comforting and hearty meal!

Lamb Stew:

Ingredients:

- 2 pounds lamb stew meat, cut into bite-sized cubes
- 2 tablespoons vegetable oil
- 1 onion, chopped
- 3 cloves garlic, minced
- 4 cups beef or lamb broth
- 1 cup red wine
- 2 tablespoons tomato paste
- 1 tablespoon Worcestershire sauce
- 1 bay leaf
- 1 teaspoon dried rosemary
- 1 teaspoon dried thyme
- 4 carrots, peeled and sliced
- 4 potatoes, peeled and diced
- 1 cup frozen peas
- Salt and black pepper to taste
- Chopped fresh parsley for garnish

Instructions:

1. In a large pot or Dutch oven, heat vegetable oil over medium-high heat. Add the lamb stew meat and brown on all sides. Remove the lamb and set it aside.
2. In the same pot, add chopped onion and sauté until softened, about 5 minutes. Add minced garlic and cook for an additional 1-2 minutes.
3. Pour in beef or lamb broth and red wine, scraping the bottom of the pot to release any flavorful bits.
4. Stir in tomato paste, Worcestershire sauce, bay leaf, dried rosemary, and dried thyme.
5. Return the browned lamb to the pot and bring the mixture to a simmer. Cover and let it simmer for about 1.5 to 2 hours, or until the meat becomes tender.

6. Add sliced carrots, diced potatoes, and frozen peas to the pot. Season with salt and black pepper to taste.

7. Continue to simmer the stew for an additional 30-45 minutes, or until the vegetables are tender.

8. Taste and adjust the seasoning if needed.

9. Discard the bay leaf.

10. Ladle the lamb stew into bowls.

11. Garnish with chopped fresh parsley.

12. Serve the lamb stew hot, and savor the rich and savory flavors!

Chicken and Vegetable Stew:

Ingredients:

- 1.5 pounds boneless, skinless chicken thighs or breasts, cut into bite-sized pieces
- 2 tablespoons olive oil
- 1 onion, chopped
- 3 cloves garlic, minced
- 4 cups chicken broth
- 1 cup white wine (optional)
- 2 tablespoons tomato paste
- 1 bay leaf
- 1 teaspoon dried thyme
- 1 teaspoon dried rosemary
- 4 carrots, peeled and sliced
- 4 potatoes, peeled and diced
- 2 cups green beans, trimmed and cut into bite-sized pieces
- 1 cup frozen peas
- Salt and black pepper to taste
- Chopped fresh parsley for garnish

Instructions:

1. In a large pot or Dutch oven, heat olive oil over medium-high heat. Add the chicken pieces and brown on all sides. Remove the chicken and set it aside.
2. In the same pot, add chopped onion and sauté until softened, about 5 minutes. Add minced garlic and cook for an additional 1-2 minutes.
3. Pour in chicken broth and white wine (if using), scraping the bottom of the pot to release any flavorful bits.
4. Stir in tomato paste, bay leaf, dried thyme, and dried rosemary.
5. Return the browned chicken to the pot and bring the mixture to a simmer. Cover and let it simmer for about 20-30 minutes, or until the chicken is cooked through.
6. Add sliced carrots, diced potatoes, green beans, and frozen peas to the pot. Season with salt and black pepper to taste.
7. Continue to simmer the stew for an additional 20-30 minutes, or until the vegetables are tender.
8. Taste and adjust the seasoning if needed.
9. Discard the bay leaf.
10. Ladle the chicken and vegetable stew into bowls.
11. Garnish with chopped fresh parsley.
12. Serve the stew hot, and relish the wholesome combination of chicken and vibrant vegetables!

Seafood Stew:

Ingredients:

- 1 pound mixed seafood (shrimp, mussels, clams, calamari, and/or white fish), cleaned and prepared
- 2 tablespoons olive oil
- 1 onion, finely chopped
- 3 cloves garlic, minced
- 1 bell pepper, diced
- 1 carrot, peeled and sliced

- 1 celery stalk, sliced
- 1 can (14 oz) diced tomatoes
- 1 cup dry white wine
- 4 cups fish or seafood broth
- 1 bay leaf
- 1 teaspoon dried thyme
- 1 teaspoon paprika
- Salt and black pepper to taste
- Pinch of saffron threads (optional)
- Fresh parsley for garnish
- Crusty bread for serving

Instructions:

1. In a large pot or Dutch oven, heat olive oil over medium heat. Add chopped onion and sauté until softened, about 5 minutes.
2. Stir in minced garlic, diced bell pepper, sliced carrot, and sliced celery. Cook for an additional 5-7 minutes until the vegetables are tender.
3. Pour in diced tomatoes (with their juice) and white wine. Simmer for 5 minutes to allow the alcohol to cook off.
4. Add fish or seafood broth, bay leaf, dried thyme, paprika, salt, black pepper, and saffron threads (if using). Mix well.
5. Bring the mixture to a simmer, then reduce the heat to low and let it simmer for about 15-20 minutes to allow the flavors to meld.
6. Add the mixed seafood to the pot and cook until the seafood is cooked through. Be careful not to overcook the seafood.
7. Taste and adjust the seasoning if needed.
8. Discard the bay leaf.
9. Ladle the seafood stew into bowls.
10. Garnish with chopped fresh parsley.
11. Serve the seafood stew hot, accompanied by crusty bread for dipping.

Turkey and Sweet Potato Stew:

Ingredients:

- 1 pound ground turkey
- 2 tablespoons olive oil
- 1 onion, chopped
- 3 cloves garlic, minced
- 2 sweet potatoes, peeled and diced
- 4 cups chicken or vegetable broth
- 1 can (14 oz) diced tomatoes
- 1 can (15 oz) black beans, drained and rinsed
- 1 teaspoon ground cumin
- 1 teaspoon chili powder
- 1/2 teaspoon paprika
- 1/2 teaspoon dried thyme
- Salt and black pepper to taste
- 1 cup corn kernels (fresh, frozen, or canned)
- 2 cups kale or spinach, chopped
- Fresh cilantro for garnish
- Lime wedges for serving

Instructions:

1. In a large pot, brown the ground turkey over medium heat. Break it apart into crumbles as it cooks. Once browned, remove any excess fat.
2. In the same pot, add olive oil and chopped onion. Sauté until the onion is softened, about 5 minutes.
3. Stir in minced garlic and cook for an additional 1-2 minutes until fragrant.
4. Add diced sweet potatoes, chicken or vegetable broth, diced tomatoes (with their juice), black beans, ground cumin, chili powder, paprika, dried thyme, salt, and black pepper. Mix well.

5. Bring the stew to a simmer, cover, and let it cook for about 15-20 minutes or until the sweet potatoes are tender.

6. Add corn kernels and chopped kale or spinach to the pot. Simmer for an additional 5 minutes until the greens are wilted.

7. Taste the stew and adjust the seasoning if needed.

8. Ladle the turkey and sweet potato stew into bowls.

9. Garnish with fresh cilantro.

10. Serve the stew hot, with lime wedges on the side for a burst of citrus flavor.

Mushroom and Barley Stew:

Ingredients:

- 1 cup pearl barley, rinsed and drained
- 2 tablespoons olive oil
- 1 onion, finely chopped
- 3 cloves garlic, minced
- 1 pound mushrooms (cremini or white), sliced
- 2 carrots, peeled and diced
- 2 celery stalks, diced
- 4 cups vegetable or mushroom broth
- 1 bay leaf
- 1 teaspoon dried thyme
- Salt and black pepper to taste
- 1 can (14 oz) diced tomatoes
- 1 tablespoon soy sauce
- Fresh parsley for garnish

Instructions:

1. In a medium saucepan, combine the rinsed barley with 3 cups of water. Bring to a boil, then reduce the heat, cover, and simmer for 30-40 minutes or until the barley is tender. Drain any excess water.

2. In a large pot, heat olive oil over medium heat. Add chopped onion and sauté until softened, about 5 minutes.

3. Stir in minced garlic and sliced mushrooms. Cook until the mushrooms release their moisture and become golden brown.

4. Add diced carrots and celery to the pot. Sauté for an additional 5-7 minutes until the vegetables are softened.

5. Pour in vegetable or mushroom broth, and add the bay leaf, dried thyme, salt, and black pepper. Bring the stew to a simmer.

6. Stir in cooked barley, diced tomatoes (with their juice), and soy sauce. Mix well.

7. Simmer the mushroom and barley stew for an additional 15-20 minutes, allowing the flavors to meld.

8. Taste and adjust the seasoning if needed.

9. Discard the bay leaf.

10. Ladle the stew into bowls.

11. Garnish with fresh parsley.

12. Serve the mushroom and barley stew hot, and savor the earthy and hearty goodness!

Vegetable Curry Stew:

Ingredients:

- 2 tablespoons vegetable oil
- 1 onion, chopped
- 3 cloves garlic, minced
- 1 tablespoon ginger, grated
- 2 tablespoons curry powder
- 1 teaspoon ground turmeric
- 1 teaspoon ground cumin
- 1 teaspoon paprika
- 1/2 teaspoon cayenne pepper (adjust to taste)

- 4 cups mixed vegetables (carrots, potatoes, bell peppers, peas, etc.), chopped
- 1 can (14 oz) diced tomatoes
- 1 can (14 oz) coconut milk
- 2 cups vegetable broth
- 1 cup lentils, rinsed and drained
- Salt and black pepper to taste
- Fresh cilantro for garnish
- Cooked rice or naan bread for serving

Instructions:

1. In a large pot, heat vegetable oil over medium heat. Add chopped onion and sauté until softened, about 5 minutes.
2. Stir in minced garlic and grated ginger. Cook for an additional 1-2 minutes until fragrant.
3. Add curry powder, ground turmeric, ground cumin, paprika, and cayenne pepper. Stir well to coat the onions in the spices.
4. Add mixed vegetables to the pot and cook for about 5-7 minutes until they begin to soften.
5. Pour in diced tomatoes, coconut milk, and vegetable broth. Stir in lentils.
6. Bring the vegetable curry stew to a simmer, then reduce the heat to low, cover, and let it simmer for about 20-25 minutes or until the lentils and vegetables are tender.
7. Season the stew with salt and black pepper to taste. Adjust the seasoning if needed.
8. Ladle the vegetable curry stew into bowls.
9. Garnish with fresh cilantro.
10. Serve the stew over cooked rice or with naan bread on the side.

Pork and Green Chile Stew:

Ingredients:

- 2 pounds pork shoulder, cut into bite-sized cubes

- 2 tablespoons vegetable oil
- 1 onion, chopped
- 3 cloves garlic, minced
- 2 cans (4 oz each) diced green chilies
- 1 can (14 oz) diced tomatoes
- 4 cups chicken or vegetable broth
- 2 teaspoons ground cumin
- 1 teaspoon dried oregano
- 1/2 teaspoon smoked paprika
- Salt and black pepper to taste
- 2 potatoes, peeled and diced
- 1 cup corn kernels (fresh, frozen, or canned)
- Fresh cilantro for garnish
- Lime wedges for serving

Instructions:

1. In a large pot or Dutch oven, heat vegetable oil over medium-high heat. Add pork cubes and brown on all sides. Remove the pork and set it aside.
2. In the same pot, add chopped onion and sauté until softened, about 5 minutes.
3. Stir in minced garlic and cook for an additional 1-2 minutes until fragrant.
4. Add diced green chilies, diced tomatoes (with their juice), chicken or vegetable broth, ground cumin, dried oregano, smoked paprika, salt, and black pepper. Mix well.
5. Return the browned pork to the pot. Bring the mixture to a simmer, cover, and let it simmer for about 1.5 to 2 hours, or until the pork is tender.
6. Add diced potatoes and corn kernels to the stew. Continue to simmer until the potatoes are cooked through.
7. Taste and adjust the seasoning if needed.
8. Ladle the pork and green chile stew into bowls.
9. Garnish with fresh cilantro.

10. Serve the stew hot, with lime wedges on the side for a burst of citrus flavor.

Black Bean and Quinoa Stew:

Ingredients:
- 1 cup quinoa, rinsed and drained
- 2 tablespoons olive oil
- 1 onion, chopped
- 3 cloves garlic, minced
- 1 bell pepper, diced
- 2 carrots, peeled and diced
- 2 celery stalks, diced
- 2 cans (15 oz each) black beans, drained and rinsed
- 1 can (14 oz) diced tomatoes
- 4 cups vegetable broth
- 1 teaspoon ground cumin
- 1 teaspoon chili powder
- 1/2 teaspoon smoked paprika
- 1/2 teaspoon dried oregano
- Salt and black pepper to taste
- 2 cups kale or spinach, chopped
- Juice of 1 lime
- Fresh cilantro for garnish
- Avocado slices for serving (optional)

Instructions:
1. In a medium saucepan, combine the rinsed quinoa with 2 cups of water. Bring to a boil, then reduce the heat, cover, and simmer for 15-20 minutes or until the quinoa is cooked and water is absorbed.
2. In a large pot, heat olive oil over medium heat. Add chopped onion and sauté until softened, about 5 minutes.
3. Stir in minced garlic, diced bell pepper, diced carrots, and diced celery. Cook for an additional 5-7 minutes until the vegetables are softened.
4. Add black beans, diced tomatoes (with their juice), vegetable broth, ground cumin, chili powder, smoked paprika, dried oregano, salt, and black pepper. Mix well.
5. Bring the stew to a simmer, then reduce the heat to low and let it simmer for about 15-20 minutes to allow the flavors to meld.

6. Stir in cooked quinoa and chopped kale or spinach. Simmer for an additional 5 minutes until the greens are wilted.
7. Squeeze lime juice into the stew and mix well.
8. Taste and adjust the seasoning if needed.
9. Ladle the black bean and quinoa stew into bowls.
10. Garnish with fresh cilantro.
11. Optionally, serve with avocado slices on top.
12. Enjoy this wholesome and protein-packed black bean and quinoa stew!

Sardine and Tomato Stew:

Ingredients:

- 2 cans (4.4 oz each) sardines in olive oil
- 2 tablespoons olive oil
- 1 onion, chopped
- 3 cloves garlic, minced
- 1 can (14 oz) diced tomatoes
- 1/2 cup tomato sauce
- 1 teaspoon dried oregano
- 1/2 teaspoon dried basil
- 1/2 teaspoon red pepper flakes (adjust to taste)
- Salt and black pepper to taste
- 1/4 cup Kalamata olives, sliced
- 2 tablespoons capers, drained
- Fresh parsley for garnish
- Cooked rice or crusty bread for serving

Instructions:

1. In a large skillet, heat olive oil over medium heat. Add chopped onion and sauté until softened, about 5 minutes.
2. Stir in minced garlic and cook for an additional 1-2 minutes until fragrant.
3. Add diced tomatoes (with their juice), tomato sauce, dried oregano, dried basil, red pepper flakes, salt, and black pepper. Mix well.

4. Simmer the tomato mixture for about 10-15 minutes, allowing the flavors to meld and the sauce to thicken.
5. Drain the olive oil from the cans of sardines, reserving a little for added flavor.
6. Gently add the sardines to the skillet, being careful not to break them apart. Simmer for an additional 5 minutes.
7. Stir in sliced Kalamata olives and capers. Simmer for a few more minutes.
8. Taste and adjust the seasoning if needed.
9. Ladle the sardine and tomato stew into bowls.
10. Garnish with fresh parsley.
11. Serve the stew hot, over cooked rice or with crusty bread on the side.

Chicken and Lentil Stew:

Ingredients:

- 1.5 pounds boneless, skinless chicken thighs or breasts, cut into bite-sized pieces
- 2 tablespoons olive oil
- 1 onion, chopped
- 3 cloves garlic, minced
- 1 cup dried brown lentils, rinsed and drained
- 4 cups chicken broth
- 1 can (14 oz) diced tomatoes
- 2 carrots, peeled and sliced
- 2 celery stalks, diced
- 1 teaspoon ground cumin
- 1 teaspoon ground coriander
- 1/2 teaspoon smoked paprika
- 1 bay leaf
- Salt and black pepper to taste
- Fresh parsley for garnish
- Lemon wedges for serving

Instructions:

1. In a large pot or Dutch oven, heat olive oil over medium-high heat. Add chicken pieces and brown on all sides. Remove the chicken and set it aside.
2. In the same pot, add chopped onion and sauté until softened, about 5 minutes.
3. Stir in minced garlic and cook for an additional 1-2 minutes until fragrant.
4. Add rinsed lentils, chicken broth, diced tomatoes (with their juice), sliced carrots, diced celery, ground cumin, ground coriander, smoked paprika, bay leaf, salt, and black pepper. Mix well.
5. Return the browned chicken to the pot. Bring the mixture to a simmer, cover, and let it simmer for about 30-40 minutes or until the lentils and chicken are cooked through.
6. Taste and adjust the seasoning if needed.
7. Discard the bay leaf.
8. Ladle the chicken and lentil stew into bowls.
9. Garnish with fresh parsley.
10. Serve the stew hot, with lemon wedges on the side for a zesty touch.

Sweet Potato and Bison Stew:

Ingredients:

- 1 pound bison stew meat, cut into bite-sized cubes
- 2 tablespoons olive oil
- 1 onion, chopped
- 3 cloves garlic, minced
- 2 sweet potatoes, peeled and diced
- 4 cups beef or bison broth
- 1 can (14 oz) diced tomatoes
- 2 carrots, peeled and sliced
- 2 celery stalks, diced
- 1 teaspoon dried thyme

- 1 teaspoon dried rosemary
- Salt and black pepper to taste
- 1 bay leaf
- 1 cup frozen peas
- Fresh parsley for garnish

Instructions:

1. In a large pot or Dutch oven, heat olive oil over medium-high heat. Add bison stew meat and brown on all sides. Remove the bison and set it aside.
2. In the same pot, add chopped onion and sauté until softened, about 5 minutes.
3. Stir in minced garlic and cook for an additional 1-2 minutes until fragrant.
4. Add diced sweet potatoes, beef or bison broth, diced tomatoes (with their juice), sliced carrots, diced celery, dried thyme, dried rosemary, salt, and black pepper. Mix well.
5. Return the browned bison to the pot. Add the bay leaf. Bring the mixture to a simmer, cover, and let it simmer for about 1.5 to 2 hours, or until the bison is tender.
6. Add frozen peas to the stew and simmer for an additional 5-7 minutes.
7. Taste and adjust the seasoning if needed.
8. Discard the bay leaf.
9. Ladle the sweet potato and bison stew into bowls.
10. Garnish with fresh parsley.
11. Serve the stew hot, and savor the rich and earthy flavors!

CHAPTER 7: PROTEIN-PACKED MAIN COURSES

Grilled Salmon:

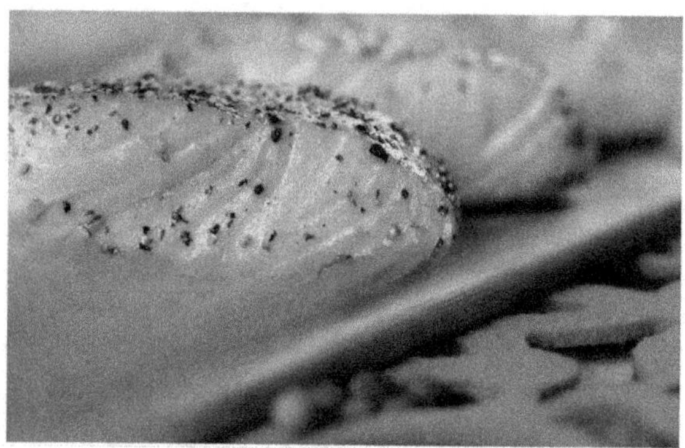

Ingredients:

- 4 salmon fillets
- 2 tablespoons olive oil
- 2 tablespoons soy sauce
- 1 tablespoon Dijon mustard
- 2 cloves garlic, minced
- 1 teaspoon honey
- 1 teaspoon lemon juice
- Salt and pepper to taste
- Lemon wedges for serving

Instructions:

1. Preheat the grill to medium-high heat.
2. In a small bowl, whisk together olive oil, soy sauce, Dijon mustard, minced garlic, honey, lemon juice, salt, and pepper to create the marinade.

3. Place the salmon fillets in a shallow dish and pour the marinade over them, ensuring each fillet is well-coated. Let it marinate for at least 15-30 minutes, allowing the flavors to infuse.

4. Remove the salmon from the marinade and discard the marinade.

5. Place the salmon fillets on the preheated grill, skin-side down. Grill for 4-6 minutes per side, or until the salmon is cooked to your liking. Use a spatula to carefully flip the fillets.

6. While grilling, baste the salmon with any remaining marinade to enhance the flavor.

7. Once the salmon is cooked through and has a nice grill mark, remove it from the grill.

8. Serve the grilled salmon hot, garnished with lemon wedges.

Bison Burger:

Ingredients:

- 1 pound ground bison
- 1/4 cup finely chopped onion
- 1 clove garlic, minced
- 1 tablespoon Worcestershire sauce
- 1 teaspoon Dijon mustard
- Salt and pepper to taste
- 4 whole wheat burger buns
- Toppings of your choice (lettuce, tomato, cheese, etc.)

Instructions:

1. In a mixing bowl, combine ground bison, chopped onion, minced garlic, Worcestershire sauce, Dijon mustard, salt, and pepper. Gently mix until all ingredients are evenly distributed.

2. Divide the mixture into four equal portions and shape them into burger patties.

3. Preheat your grill or stovetop grilling pan over medium-high heat.

4. Place the bison patties on the preheated grill or pan. Cook for about 4-5 minutes per side for medium doneness or adjust based on your preference.

5. Toast the whole wheat burger buns on the grill for a minute or until they are lightly golden.

6. Assemble your bison burgers by placing each patty on a bun and adding your favorite toppings, such as lettuce, tomato, and cheese.

7. Serve the bison burgers hot and enjoy with your preferred side dishes.

Turkey Stir-Fry:

Ingredients:

- 1 pound turkey breast, thinly sliced
- 2 tablespoons soy sauce
- 1 tablespoon oyster sauce
- 1 tablespoon hoisin sauce
- 1 teaspoon sesame oil
- 2 tablespoons vegetable oil
- 1 onion, thinly sliced
- 1 bell pepper, thinly sliced
- 1 cup broccoli florets
- 2 carrots, julienned
- 2 cloves garlic, minced
- 1 teaspoon ginger, grated
- 3 green onions, sliced
- Cooked rice or noodles for serving

Instructions:

1. In a bowl, combine soy sauce, oyster sauce, hoisin sauce, and sesame oil. Mix well to create the sauce for the stir-fry.

2. Heat vegetable oil in a wok or large skillet over medium-high heat.

3. Add thinly sliced turkey to the hot pan and stir-fry for 2-3 minutes or until the turkey is cooked through.

4. Remove the cooked turkey from the pan and set it aside.

5. In the same pan, add a bit more oil if needed. Stir in sliced onion, bell pepper, broccoli, and julienned carrots. Cook for 3-4 minutes until the vegetables are slightly tender but still crisp.

6. Add minced garlic and grated ginger to the vegetables, stir-frying for an additional 1-2 minutes until fragrant.

7. Return the cooked turkey to the pan with the vegetables.

8. Pour the prepared sauce over the turkey and vegetables. Toss everything together until well coated and heated through.

9. Add sliced green onions and stir briefly.

10. Serve the turkey stir-fry over cooked rice or noodles.

Chicken Breast with Vegetables:

Ingredients:

- 4 boneless, skinless chicken breasts
- Salt and pepper to taste
- 2 tablespoons olive oil
- 2 cloves garlic, minced
- 1 teaspoon dried oregano
- 1 teaspoon dried thyme
- 1 teaspoon paprika
- 1 teaspoon onion powder
- 1 cup cherry tomatoes, halved
- 1 zucchini, sliced
- 1 bell pepper, sliced
- 1 cup broccoli florets
- 1/4 cup chicken broth

- Fresh parsley for garnish

Instructions:

1. Preheat your oven to 375°F (190°C).
2. Season the chicken breasts with salt, pepper, dried oregano, dried thyme, paprika, and onion powder on both sides.
3. In an oven-safe skillet, heat olive oil over medium-high heat. Add the seasoned chicken breasts and sear them for 2-3 minutes on each side until golden brown.
4. Remove the seared chicken from the skillet and set it aside.
5. In the same skillet, add minced garlic and sauté for about 1 minute until fragrant.
6. Add cherry tomatoes, zucchini, bell pepper, and broccoli to the skillet. Cook the vegetables for 3-4 minutes until they begin to soften.
7. Pour chicken broth into the skillet and stir, scraping any browned bits from the bottom.
8. Return the seared chicken breasts to the skillet, nestling them among the vegetables.
9. Transfer the skillet to the preheated oven and bake for 20-25 minutes or until the chicken is cooked through.
10. Garnish with fresh parsley before serving.

Tofu and Broccoli Stir-Fry:

Ingredients:

- 1 block (14 oz) firm tofu, pressed and cubed
- 3 tablespoons soy sauce
- 1 tablespoon hoisin sauce
- 1 tablespoon rice vinegar
- 1 tablespoon sesame oil
- 1 tablespoon cornstarch
- 2 tablespoons vegetable oil
- 3 cups broccoli florets

- 1 red bell pepper, thinly sliced
- 2 carrots, julienned
- 3 cloves garlic, minced
- 1 teaspoon ginger, grated
- Cooked rice or noodles for serving
- Sesame seeds and green onions for garnish

Instructions:

1. In a bowl, mix soy sauce, hoisin sauce, rice vinegar, sesame oil, and cornstarch to create the sauce for the stir-fry.
2. Heat 1 tablespoon of vegetable oil in a wok or large skillet over medium-high heat.
3. Add cubed tofu to the hot pan and stir-fry for 5-7 minutes, or until the tofu is golden brown. Remove tofu from the pan and set it aside.
4. In the same pan, add the remaining tablespoon of oil. Stir in minced garlic and grated ginger, cooking for about 1 minute until fragrant.
5. Add broccoli florets, sliced red bell pepper, and julienned carrots to the pan. Stir-fry for 3-4 minutes until the vegetables are slightly tender but still crisp.
6. Return the cooked tofu to the pan with the vegetables.
7. Pour the prepared sauce over the tofu and vegetables. Toss everything together until well coated and heated through.
8. Serve the tofu and broccoli stir-fry over cooked rice or noodles.

Lentil and Quinoa Bowl:

Ingredients:

- 1 cup dry quinoa, rinsed
- 1/2 cup dry green or brown lentils, rinsed
- 2 1/2 cups vegetable broth or water
- 1 tablespoon olive oil
- 1 onion, finely chopped
- 2 cloves garlic, minced
- 1 bell pepper, diced
- 1 zucchini, diced

- 1 carrot, grated
- 1 teaspoon ground cumin
- 1 teaspoon smoked paprika
- Salt and pepper to taste
- Juice of 1 lemon
- Fresh parsley or cilantro for garnish

Instructions:

1. In a medium saucepan, combine quinoa, lentils, and vegetable broth or water. Bring to a boil, then reduce heat to low, cover, and simmer for 15-20 minutes or until quinoa and lentils are cooked and water is absorbed.
2. While the quinoa and lentils are cooking, heat olive oil in a large skillet over medium heat.
3. Add chopped onion and minced garlic to the skillet, sautéing for 2-3 minutes until softened.
4. Stir in diced bell pepper, zucchini, and grated carrot. Cook for an additional 5-7 minutes until the vegetables are tender but still crisp.
5. Add ground cumin, smoked paprika, salt, and pepper to the vegetables. Mix well to combine.
6. Once the quinoa and lentils are cooked, fluff them with a fork and add them to the skillet with the sautéed vegetables. Stir to combine.
7. Squeeze the juice of one lemon over the mixture and toss everything together.
8. Adjust salt and pepper to taste.
9. Serve the lentil and quinoa mixture in bowls, garnished with fresh parsley or cilantro.

Grilled Bison Steak:

Ingredients:

- 2 bison sirloin or ribeye steaks (about 8 ounces each)
- 2 tablespoons olive oil
- 2 teaspoons dried rosemary
- 1 teaspoon garlic powder
- 1 teaspoon onion powder
- 1 teaspoon paprika
- Salt and pepper to taste

Instructions:

1. Preheat your grill to medium-high heat.
2. In a small bowl, mix olive oil, dried rosemary, garlic powder, onion powder, paprika, salt, and pepper to create a seasoning paste.
3. Pat the bison steaks dry with a paper towel.
4. Brush the steaks with the seasoning paste on both sides, ensuring they are evenly coated.
5. Place the seasoned bison steaks on the preheated grill. Grill for approximately 4-5 minutes per side for medium-rare, adjusting the time based on your preferred level of doneness.
6. Use tongs to carefully flip the steaks halfway through the cooking time.
7. Allow the grilled bison steaks to rest for a few minutes before slicing.
8. Slice the steaks against the grain and serve immediately.

Shrimp and Asparagus:

Ingredients:

- 1 pound large shrimp, peeled and deveined
- 1 bunch asparagus, trimmed and cut into bite-sized pieces
- 2 tablespoons olive oil
- 3 cloves garlic, minced
- 1 teaspoon lemon zest
- 2 tablespoons lemon juice
- 1 teaspoon dried oregano
- Salt and pepper to taste
- Crushed red pepper flakes (optional)
- Fresh parsley for garnish

Instructions:

1. In a bowl, mix shrimp with olive oil, minced garlic, lemon zest, lemon juice, dried oregano, salt, and pepper. Let it marinate for about 15-30 minutes.

2. Heat a large skillet over medium-high heat.

3. Add the marinated shrimp to the skillet, spreading them out in a single layer. Cook for 2-3 minutes on one side until they start to turn pink.

4. Flip the shrimp and add the asparagus to the skillet. Cook for an additional 3-4 minutes or until the shrimp are fully cooked, and the asparagus is tender-crisp.

5. Adjust seasoning to taste and add optional crushed red pepper flakes for a bit of heat.

6. Garnish with fresh parsley before serving.

7. Serve the shrimp and asparagus over rice, pasta, or enjoy it on its own.

Beef and Vegetable Skewers:

Ingredients:

- 1 pound beef sirloin or tenderloin, cut into bite-sized cubes
- 1 red bell pepper, cut into chunks
- 1 green bell pepper, cut into chunks
- 1 zucchini, sliced into rounds
- 1 red onion, cut into chunks
- 8-10 cherry tomatoes
- 3 tablespoons olive oil
- 2 tablespoons soy sauce
- 2 tablespoons balsamic vinegar
- 2 cloves garlic, minced
- 1 teaspoon dried oregano
- Salt and pepper to taste
- Wooden skewers, soaked in water for 30 minutes

Instructions:

1. In a bowl, mix olive oil, soy sauce, balsamic vinegar, minced garlic, dried oregano, salt, and pepper to create the marinade.

2. Thread the beef cubes, bell peppers, zucchini slices, red onion chunks, and cherry tomatoes onto the soaked wooden skewers, alternating between the ingredients.

3. Place the assembled skewers in a shallow dish and brush them with the marinade, ensuring they are well-coated. Let them marinate for at least 30 minutes.

4. Preheat your grill or grill pan over medium-high heat.

5. Grill the beef and vegetable skewers for about 8-10 minutes, turning occasionally, until the beef is cooked to your liking and the vegetables are tender with a slight char.

6. Brush the skewers with additional marinade while grilling for extra flavor.

7. Once cooked, remove the skewers from the grill and let them rest for a few minutes.

8. Serve the beef and vegetable skewers hot, either as an appetizer or over a bed of rice or quinoa.

Salmon Salad:

Ingredients:

- 2 salmon fillets
- Salt and pepper to taste
- 2 tablespoons olive oil
- 6 cups mixed salad greens (e.g., spinach, arugula, or mixed greens)
- 1 cucumber, sliced
- 1 cup cherry tomatoes, halved
- 1/4 red onion, thinly sliced
- 1/4 cup Kalamata olives, pitted and sliced
- 1/4 cup feta cheese, crumbled
- Lemon wedges for serving

For the dressing:

- 3 tablespoons olive oil
- 1 tablespoon balsamic vinegar

- 1 teaspoon Dijon mustard
- 1 clove garlic, minced
- Salt and pepper to taste

Instructions:

1. Preheat your oven to 400°F (200°C).
2. Season the salmon fillets with salt and pepper. Place them on a baking sheet and drizzle with olive oil.
3. Bake the salmon in the preheated oven for 12-15 minutes, or until the salmon is cooked through and flakes easily with a fork.
4. While the salmon is baking, prepare the salad. In a large bowl, combine the mixed salad greens, sliced cucumber, cherry tomatoes, red onion, Kalamata olives, and crumbled feta cheese.
5. In a small bowl, whisk together the ingredients for the dressing: olive oil, balsamic vinegar, Dijon mustard, minced garlic, salt, and pepper.
6. Once the salmon is done, remove it from the oven and let it cool slightly.
7. Flake the salmon into bite-sized pieces and add it to the salad.
8. Drizzle the salad with the prepared dressing and toss everything gently to combine.
9. Serve the salmon salad on plates, garnishing with additional feta cheese and lemon wedges if desired.

Eggplant and Ground Lamb:

Ingredients:

- 1 large eggplant, diced
- 1 pound ground lamb
- 1 onion, finely chopped
- 3 cloves garlic, minced
- 1 can (14 oz) diced tomatoes
- 2 tablespoons tomato paste

- 1 teaspoon dried oregano
- 1 teaspoon ground cumin
- 1/2 teaspoon cinnamon
- Salt and pepper to taste
- 2 tablespoons olive oil
- Fresh parsley for garnish

Instructions:

1. In a large skillet, heat olive oil over medium-high heat.
2. Add chopped onion and minced garlic to the skillet, sautéing for 2-3 minutes until softened.
3. Add ground lamb to the skillet and cook until browned, breaking it apart with a spoon as it cooks.
4. Stir in diced eggplant and continue cooking for another 5-7 minutes until the eggplant starts to soften.
5. Add diced tomatoes, tomato paste, dried oregano, ground cumin, cinnamon, salt, and pepper to the skillet. Mix well.
6. Reduce the heat to medium-low, cover the skillet, and simmer for 15-20 minutes, allowing the flavors to meld and the eggplant to become tender.
7. Adjust seasoning to taste.
8. Garnish with fresh parsley before serving.

Pork Tenderloin with Apples:

Ingredients:

- 1.5 to 2 pounds pork tenderloin
- Salt and pepper to taste
- 2 tablespoons olive oil
- 2 apples, cored and sliced (such as Granny Smith or Honeycrisp)
- 1 onion, thinly sliced
- 2 cloves garlic, minced

- 1 teaspoon dried thyme
- 1/2 cup apple cider or apple juice
- 1/2 cup chicken broth
- 2 tablespoons Dijon mustard
- 2 tablespoons maple syrup
- Fresh parsley for garnish

Instructions:

1. Preheat your oven to 375°F (190°C).
2. Season the pork tenderloin with salt and pepper.
3. In an oven-safe skillet, heat olive oil over medium-high heat.
4. Sear the pork tenderloin on all sides until browned, about 2-3 minutes per side.
5. Remove the pork from the skillet and set it aside.
6. In the same skillet, add sliced apples and onions. Cook for 3-4 minutes until softened.
7. Add minced garlic and dried thyme to the skillet, sautéing for an additional 1-2 minutes until fragrant.
8. Place the seared pork tenderloin back into the skillet among the apples and onions.
9. In a bowl, whisk together apple cider or juice, chicken broth, Dijon mustard, and maple syrup. Pour this mixture over the pork and apples.
10. Transfer the skillet to the preheated oven and roast for about 20-25 minutes or until the internal temperature of the pork reaches 145°F (63°C).
11. Once done, let the pork rest for a few minutes before slicing.
12. Garnish with fresh parsley before serving.

Quinoa and Black Bean Stuffed Bell Peppers:

Ingredients:

- 4 large bell peppers, halved and seeds removed
- 1 cup quinoa, rinsed
- 2 cups vegetable broth or water

- 1 can (15 oz) black beans, drained and rinsed
- 1 cup corn kernels (fresh or frozen)
- 1 cup diced tomatoes
- 1 cup diced red onion
- 1 teaspoon ground cumin
- 1 teaspoon chili powder
- Salt and pepper to taste
- 1 cup shredded cheddar or Mexican blend cheese (optional)
- Fresh cilantro for garnish

Instructions:

1. Preheat your oven to 375°F (190°C).
2. In a medium saucepan, bring the vegetable broth or water to a boil. Add quinoa, reduce heat to low, cover, and simmer for 15-20 minutes or until quinoa is cooked and liquid is absorbed.
3. In a large mixing bowl, combine cooked quinoa, black beans, corn, diced tomatoes, diced red onion, ground cumin, chili powder, salt, and pepper. Mix well.
4. Place the halved bell peppers in a baking dish.
5. Stuff each bell pepper half with the quinoa and black bean mixture, pressing it down gently.
6. If desired, sprinkle shredded cheese over the top of each stuffed pepper.
7. Cover the baking dish with foil and bake in the preheated oven for 25-30 minutes or until the bell peppers are tender.
8. Remove the foil and bake for an additional 5-10 minutes, allowing the cheese to melt and become golden brown.
9. Garnish the stuffed bell peppers with fresh cilantro before serving.

Steamed Broccoli:

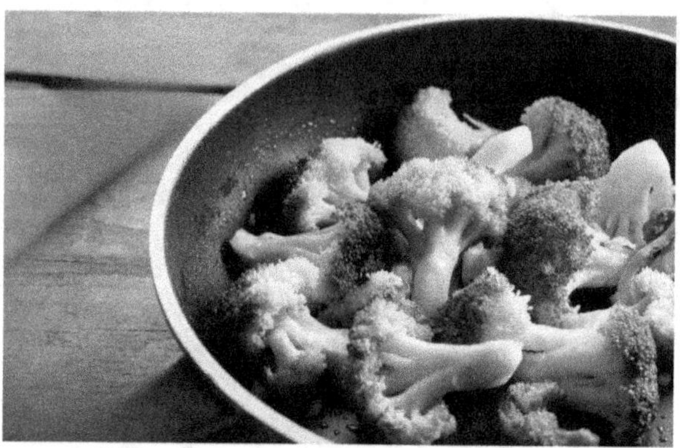

Ingredients:

- Fresh broccoli florets
- Water for steaming
- Salt (optional)
- Olive oil or butter (optional)

Instructions:

1. Wash the broccoli thoroughly under cold running water.
2. Cut the broccoli into bite-sized florets, ensuring they are relatively uniform in size for even steaming.
3. Fill a pot or a steamer with about an inch of water. Place a steamer basket or a colander above the water level, making sure the broccoli won't touch the water.
4. Bring the water to a boil over medium-high heat.
5. Add the broccoli florets to the steamer basket, spreading them out to allow for even steaming.

6. Cover the pot or steamer with a lid and reduce the heat to maintain a gentle simmer.

7. Steam the broccoli for 5-7 minutes or until it reaches your desired level of tenderness. Be cautious not to overcook, as you want the broccoli to remain crisp and vibrant.

8. Once done, remove the broccoli from the steamer and transfer it to a serving dish.

9. If desired, season the steamed broccoli with a pinch of salt and drizzle with olive oil or melted butter for added flavor.

10. Serve the steamed broccoli as a nutritious side dish alongside your favorite main course.

Roasted Sweet Potatoes:

Ingredients:

- Sweet potatoes
- Olive oil
- Salt
- Pepper
- Optional: Herbs or spices of your choice (e.g., rosemary, thyme, paprika)

Instructions:

1. Preheat your oven to 400°F (200°C).

2. Wash and peel the sweet potatoes. Cut them into evenly sized cubes or wedges.

3. Place the sweet potato pieces in a large mixing bowl.

4. Drizzle olive oil over the sweet potatoes, ensuring they are well-coated. Toss the sweet potatoes to evenly distribute the oil.

5. Season the sweet potatoes with salt and pepper to taste. Add any optional herbs or spices at this point.

6. Spread the sweet potato pieces in a single layer on a baking sheet lined with parchment paper or lightly greased.

7. Place the baking sheet in the preheated oven and roast for about 25-30 minutes or until the sweet potatoes are golden brown and tender. Be sure to toss or flip the sweet potatoes halfway through the roasting time for even cooking.

8. Once roasted to perfection, remove the sweet potatoes from the oven.

9. Allow them to cool slightly before serving.

10. Serve the roasted sweet potatoes as a delightful side dish or a healthy snack.

Sautéed Spinach:

Ingredients:

- Fresh spinach leaves, washed and trimmed
- Olive oil or butter
- Garlic cloves, minced (optional)
- Salt and pepper to taste
- Lemon juice (optional)

Instructions:

1. Heat a large skillet or pan over medium heat.

2. Add a drizzle of olive oil or a knob of butter to the pan.

3. If using, add minced garlic to the heated oil or butter. Sauté for about 30 seconds until fragrant but not browned.

4. Add the fresh spinach leaves to the pan. You may need to do this in batches, depending on the size of your pan, as spinach cooks down significantly.

5. Gently toss the spinach with tongs or a spatula as it wilts. This should take 2-3 minutes.

6. Season the sautéed spinach with salt and pepper to taste. Adjust the seasoning according to your preference.

7. If desired, squeeze a bit of lemon juice over the spinach for a touch of brightness.

8. Continue tossing and cooking until the spinach is fully wilted and tender.

9. Once done, remove the sautéed spinach from the heat immediately to prevent overcooking.

10. Serve the sautéed spinach as a flavorful and nutritious side dish.

Grilled Asparagus:

Ingredients:

- Fresh asparagus spears, trimmed
- Olive oil
- Salt and pepper to taste
- Optional: Lemon zest or balsamic vinegar for added flavor

Instructions:

1. Preheat your grill to medium-high heat.
2. Wash and trim the tough ends from the asparagus spears.
3. In a large bowl, toss the asparagus with olive oil, ensuring they are evenly coated.
4. Season the asparagus with salt and pepper to taste. You can also add optional lemon zest or a splash of balsamic vinegar for extra flavor.
5. Place the asparagus spears directly on the preheated grill grates.
6. Grill the asparagus for 4-6 minutes, turning occasionally, until they are tender with a slight char.
7. Keep a close eye on the asparagus to prevent overcooking; they should remain crisp-tender.
8. Once grilled to perfection, remove the asparagus from the grill.
9. Serve the grilled asparagus as a delightful side dish to complement your main course.

Cauliflower Mash:

Ingredients:

- 1 head of cauliflower, washed and cut into florets
- 2 cloves garlic, minced
- 2 tablespoons butter or olive oil
- 1/4 cup milk or vegetable broth (adjust for desired consistency)

- Salt and pepper to taste
- Optional: Fresh herbs (e.g., thyme or chives) for garnish

Instructions:

1. Steam or boil the cauliflower florets until they are tender. This usually takes about 10-15 minutes.
2. Drain the cauliflower well to remove excess moisture.
3. In a blender or food processor, combine the cooked cauliflower, minced garlic, butter or olive oil, and a pinch of salt and pepper.
4. Blend the ingredients until smooth and creamy. You may need to stop and scrape down the sides of the blender or processor to ensure everything is well combined.
5. Add the milk or vegetable broth gradually, blending continuously, until you achieve your desired consistency.
6. Taste the cauliflower mash and adjust the seasoning as needed.
7. Transfer the mashed cauliflower to a serving bowl.
8. If desired, garnish with fresh herbs like thyme or chives.
9. Serve the cauliflower mash as a tasty and lower-carb alternative to traditional mashed potatoes.

Balsamic Glazed Brussels Sprouts:

Ingredients:

- 1 pound Brussels sprouts, trimmed and halved
- 2 tablespoons olive oil
- 2 tablespoons balsamic vinegar
- 1 tablespoon honey or maple syrup
- Salt and pepper to taste
- Optional: Grated Parmesan cheese for garnish

Instructions:

1. Preheat your oven to 400°F (200°C).

2. In a large bowl, toss the halved Brussels sprouts with olive oil, ensuring they are well-coated.

3. Spread the Brussels sprouts in a single layer on a baking sheet lined with parchment paper or lightly greased.

4. Roast the Brussels sprouts in the preheated oven for 20-25 minutes or until they are golden brown and crisp on the edges. Toss them halfway through the roasting time for even cooking.

5. While the Brussels sprouts are roasting, mix balsamic vinegar and honey (or maple syrup) in a small bowl.

6. Remove the Brussels sprouts from the oven and drizzle the balsamic-honey mixture over them. Toss to coat evenly.

7. Season with salt and pepper to taste. Toss again to ensure even coating.

8. Optionally, sprinkle grated Parmesan cheese over the Brussels sprouts for an extra layer of flavor.

9. Return the baking sheet to the oven and roast for an additional 5-7 minutes or until the glaze is caramelized and the Brussels sprouts are tender.

10. Once done, transfer the balsamic glazed Brussels sprouts to a serving dish.

Quinoa Salad:

Ingredients:

- 1 cup quinoa, rinsed
- 2 cups water or vegetable broth
- 1 cup cherry tomatoes, halved
- 1 cucumber, diced
- 1 bell pepper (any color), diced
- 1/4 cup red onion, finely chopped
- 1/4 cup feta cheese, crumbled
- 1/4 cup fresh parsley, chopped
- 1/4 cup olive oil

- 2 tablespoons balsamic vinegar
- 1 teaspoon Dijon mustard
- Salt and pepper to taste
- Optional: Lemon zest for a citrusy kick

Instructions:

1. In a medium saucepan, combine quinoa and water or vegetable broth. Bring to a boil, then reduce the heat to low, cover, and simmer for 15-20 minutes or until the quinoa is cooked and the liquid is absorbed.
2. Fluff the quinoa with a fork and let it cool to room temperature.
3. In a large bowl, combine the cooked quinoa, cherry tomatoes, cucumber, bell pepper, red onion, feta cheese, and fresh parsley.
4. In a small bowl or jar, whisk together olive oil, balsamic vinegar, Dijon mustard, salt, and pepper. Optionally, add lemon zest for extra flavor.
5. Pour the dressing over the quinoa mixture and toss everything together until well coated.
6. Adjust seasoning to taste.
7. Chill the quinoa salad in the refrigerator for at least 30 minutes before serving to enhance the flavors.
8. Before serving, give the salad a final toss and garnish with additional fresh parsley or feta cheese if desired.

Cucumber Salad:

Ingredients:

- 2 medium cucumbers, thinly sliced
- 1/2 red onion, thinly sliced
- 1/4 cup fresh dill, chopped
- 1/4 cup feta cheese, crumbled
- 2 tablespoons olive oil
- 2 tablespoons red wine vinegar

- 1 teaspoon honey or maple syrup
- Salt and pepper to taste

Instructions:

1. In a large bowl, combine thinly sliced cucumbers, red onion, fresh dill, and crumbled feta cheese.
2. In a small bowl, whisk together olive oil, red wine vinegar, honey or maple syrup, salt, and pepper to create the dressing.
3. Pour the dressing over the cucumber mixture.
4. Toss the salad gently to ensure the ingredients are well coated with the dressing.
5. Allow the cucumber salad to marinate in the refrigerator for at least 15-30 minutes to enhance the flavors.
6. Before serving, give the salad a final toss and adjust the seasoning if necessary.
7. Optionally, garnish with additional dill or feta cheese before serving.

Steamed Artichokes:

Ingredients:

- 2 large artichokes
- Lemon wedges (for serving)
- Optional: Melted butter, garlic aioli, or balsamic vinaigrette for dipping

Instructions:

1. Start by trimming the stem of each artichoke, leaving about 1 inch attached. Cut about 1 inch off the top of each artichoke to remove the thorny tips.
2. Rinse the artichokes under cold running water, gently spreading the leaves to remove any dirt or debris.
3. If desired, use kitchen scissors to trim the pointy tips off the outer leaves.
4. Fill a large pot with about 2 inches of water and bring it to a simmer over medium heat.
5. Place a steamer basket in the pot. Put the prepared artichokes in the basket, stem side down.

6. Cover the pot with a lid and steam the artichokes for approximately 25-40 minutes, depending on their size. They are done when a leaf near the center pulls away easily.

7. While the artichokes are steaming, you can prepare a dipping sauce if desired, such as melted butter, garlic aioli, or balsamic vinaigrette.

8. Once steamed, remove the artichokes from the pot and let them cool for a few minutes.

9. Serve the steamed artichokes with lemon wedges for squeezing over the leaves and your chosen dipping sauce.

Roasted Red Peppers:

Ingredients:

- Red bell peppers
- Olive oil
- Salt and pepper to taste
- Optional: Garlic cloves (peeled), balsamic vinegar, or herbs like thyme for added flavor

Instructions:

1. Preheat your oven to 400°F (200°C).
2. Wash and dry the red bell peppers.
3. Cut the peppers in half and remove the seeds and membranes.
4. Place the pepper halves on a baking sheet, cut side down.
5. If using, tuck peeled garlic cloves among the peppers for extra flavor.
6. Drizzle olive oil over the peppers, ensuring they are well-coated.
7. Season with salt and pepper to taste. Optionally, add balsamic vinegar or sprinkle with herbs like thyme.
8. Roast the peppers in the preheated oven for 25-30 minutes or until the skin is charred and the peppers are tender.
9. Remove the baking sheet from the oven and let the peppers cool for a few minutes.

10. Once cooled, peel off the charred skin. It should come off easily. Slice or dice the roasted red peppers as desired.

Stir-Fried Bok Choy:

Ingredients:

- 1 pound baby bok choy, washed and trimmed
- 2 tablespoons vegetable oil (such as sesame oil or peanut oil)
- 2 cloves garlic, minced
- 1 teaspoon fresh ginger, grated
- 2 tablespoons soy sauce
- 1 tablespoon oyster sauce (optional)
- 1 teaspoon sesame seeds (optional)
- Pinch of red pepper flakes (optional, for heat)
- Salt and pepper to taste

Instructions:

1. Cut the baby bok choy in half lengthwise or leave them whole if they are small.
2. Heat vegetable oil in a wok or large skillet over medium-high heat.
3. Add minced garlic and grated ginger to the hot oil, and stir-fry for about 30 seconds until fragrant.
4. Add the baby bok choy to the wok, tossing and stirring constantly with a spatula or tongs.
5. Cook the bok choy for 3-5 minutes, or until the leaves are wilted and the stems are tender-crisp. Be attentive to avoid overcooking.
6. Drizzle soy sauce and oyster sauce (if using) over the bok choy. Continue to stir-fry for an additional 1-2 minutes.
7. Season with salt and pepper to taste. Optionally, add sesame seeds and a pinch of red pepper flakes for extra flavor and heat.
8. Once the bok choy is cooked to your liking, remove it from the heat.
9. Serve the stir-fried bok choy as a tasty and nutritious side dish.

Sautéed Mushrooms:

Ingredients:

- 1 pound mushrooms, cleaned and sliced
- 2 tablespoons butter or olive oil
- 2 cloves garlic, minced
- Salt and pepper to taste
- Fresh herbs like thyme or parsley (optional)

Instructions:

1. Heat butter or olive oil in a large skillet over medium-high heat.
2. Add minced garlic to the hot oil or butter and sauté for about 30 seconds until fragrant.
3. Add the sliced mushrooms to the skillet, spreading them out in a single layer.
4. Allow the mushrooms to cook undisturbed for a couple of minutes to develop a nice golden color on one side.
5. Stir the mushrooms occasionally to ensure even cooking.
6. Sauté the mushrooms for 5-7 minutes or until they are tender and have released their moisture.
7. Season the mushrooms with salt and pepper to taste. Add fresh herbs like thyme or parsley if desired.
8. Continue to cook for an additional 2-3 minutes to allow the flavors to meld.
9. Once done, remove the sautéed mushrooms from the heat.
10. Serve as a delicious side dish, over pasta, or as a topping for steak or chicken.

Accompaniments:

Avocado Slices:

Ingredients:

- Ripe avocados
- Lime or lemon wedges (for serving)

* Salt and pepper to taste
* Optional: Red pepper flakes, chili powder, or your favorite seasoning

Instructions:

1. Cut the ripe avocados in half lengthwise and remove the pit.
2. Use a spoon to carefully scoop out avocado slices, maintaining their shape.
3. Arrange the avocado slices on a serving plate.
4. Squeeze lime or lemon juice over the avocado slices to add a fresh flavor and prevent browning.
5. Sprinkle salt and pepper to taste on the avocado slices.
6. Optionally, add a pinch of red pepper flakes, chili powder, or your favorite seasoning for an extra kick.
7. Serve the avocado slices immediately as a simple and nutritious snack or as a side dish.

Salsa:

Ingredients:

* 4 medium tomatoes, diced
* 1 small red onion, finely chopped
* 1-2 jalapeños, seeds removed and finely chopped
* 1/4 cup fresh cilantro, chopped
* 2 cloves garlic, minced
* Juice of 1 lime
* Salt and pepper to taste

Instructions:

1. In a large bowl, combine diced tomatoes, finely chopped red onion, jalapeños, cilantro, and minced garlic.
2. Squeeze the juice of one lime over the mixture.
3. Season with salt and pepper to taste.
4. Gently toss the ingredients together until well combined.

5. Let the salsa sit for at least 15-30 minutes to allow the flavors to meld.

6. Taste and adjust seasoning if necessary.

7. Serve the salsa with tortilla chips, tacos, grilled meats, or your favorite dishes.

Hummus:

Ingredients:

- 1 can (15 ounces) chickpeas (garbanzo beans), drained and rinsed
- 1/4 cup tahini (sesame paste)
- 2 tablespoons lemon juice (about 1 medium lemon)
- 2 cloves garlic, minced
- 1/2 teaspoon ground cumin
- 1/4 teaspoon paprika (plus extra for garnish)
- 1/4 cup extra-virgin olive oil
- Salt to taste
- Water (as needed for desired consistency)
- Optional: Pine nuts, chopped fresh parsley, or a drizzle of olive oil for garnish

Instructions:

1. In a food processor, combine chickpeas, tahini, lemon juice, minced garlic, ground cumin, and paprika.

2. Pulse the ingredients until well combined and the mixture starts to become smooth.

3. With the food processor running, slowly drizzle in the olive oil, blending until the hummus reaches a creamy consistency.

4. Season the hummus with salt to taste. If needed, add a bit of water while processing to achieve the desired smoothness.

5. Taste the hummus and adjust the seasoning or add more lemon juice if desired.

6. Transfer the hummus to a serving bowl.

7. Optionally, garnish with a sprinkle of paprika, pine nuts, chopped fresh parsley, or a drizzle of olive oil.

8. Serve the hummus with pita bread, vegetables, or as a tasty dip for your favorite snacks.

Tzatziki Sauce:

Ingredients:

- 1 cup Greek yogurt
- 1 cucumber, finely grated and squeezed to remove excess moisture
- 2 cloves garlic, minced
- 1 tablespoon fresh dill, chopped
- 1 tablespoon extra-virgin olive oil
- 1 teaspoon white wine vinegar or lemon juice
- Salt and pepper to taste

Instructions:

1. In a bowl, combine Greek yogurt, finely grated cucumber, minced garlic, and chopped fresh dill.
2. Add extra-virgin olive oil and white wine vinegar (or lemon juice) to the mixture.
3. Season the tzatziki sauce with salt and pepper to taste.
4. Stir the ingredients together until well combined.
5. Let the tzatziki sauce chill in the refrigerator for at least 30 minutes to allow the flavors to meld.
6. Taste and adjust seasoning if necessary before serving.
7. Serve the tzatziki sauce as a refreshing dip with pita bread, vegetables, or as a condiment for grilled meats.

Olive Tapenade:

Ingredients:

- 1 cup pitted Kalamata olives
- 1/2 cup green olives, pitted
- 2 tablespoons capers, drained

- 2 cloves garlic, minced
- 2 tablespoons fresh parsley, chopped
- 1 tablespoon fresh lemon juice
- 1/4 cup extra-virgin olive oil
- Black pepper to taste

Instructions:

1. In a food processor, combine Kalamata olives, green olives, capers, minced garlic, fresh parsley, and fresh lemon juice.
2. Pulse the ingredients until they are finely chopped and well combined.
3. With the food processor running, slowly drizzle in the extra-virgin olive oil until the tapenade reaches your desired consistency.
4. Season the olive tapenade with black pepper to taste. Remember that the olives and capers are already salty, so additional salt may not be needed.
5. Continue pulsing until the tapenade is well mixed.
6. Transfer the olive tapenade to a serving bowl.
7. Optionally, drizzle a bit of extra-virgin olive oil over the top before serving.
8. Serve the olive tapenade with crusty bread, crackers, or as a flavorful topping for grilled meats.

Guacamole:

Ingredients:

- 3 ripe avocados
- 1 small red onion, finely chopped
- 1-2 tomatoes, diced
- 1-2 cloves garlic, minced
- 1-2 jalapeños, seeds and membranes removed, finely chopped
- 1/4 cup fresh cilantro, chopped
- Juice of 2 limes
- Salt and pepper to taste

Instructions:

1. Cut the avocados in half, remove the pits, and scoop the flesh into a mixing bowl.
2. Mash the avocados with a fork or potato masher until you achieve your desired level of creaminess.
3. Add finely chopped red onion, diced tomatoes, minced garlic, chopped jalapeños, and fresh cilantro to the mashed avocados.
4. Squeeze the juice of two limes over the mixture.
5. Season the guacamole with salt and pepper to taste.
6. Gently stir all the ingredients together until well combined.
7. Taste and adjust the seasoning or lime juice if needed.
8. Optionally, add additional chopped cilantro or a dash of hot sauce for extra flavor.
9. Cover the guacamole with plastic wrap, ensuring it touches the surface to prevent browning.
10. Refrigerate for at least 30 minutes to let the flavors meld before serving.

Chimichurri Sauce:

Ingredients:

- 1 cup fresh parsley, finely chopped
- 1/4 cup fresh cilantro, finely chopped
- 3 cloves garlic, minced
- 1 teaspoon dried oregano
- 1/2 teaspoon red pepper flakes (adjust to taste)
- 1/4 cup red wine vinegar
- 1/2 cup extra-virgin olive oil
- Salt and pepper to taste

Instructions:

1. In a bowl, combine finely chopped fresh parsley, fresh cilantro, minced garlic, dried oregano, and red pepper flakes.
2. Add red wine vinegar to the mixture and stir to combine.

3. Slowly drizzle in the extra-virgin olive oil while stirring to emulsify the sauce.

4. Season the chimichurri sauce with salt and pepper to taste.

5. Taste and adjust the seasoning, vinegar, or olive oil according to your preference.

6. Let the chimichurri sauce sit for at least 15-30 minutes to allow the flavors to meld.

7. Stir the sauce before serving to ensure the ingredients are well distributed.

8. Serve the chimichurri sauce as a flavorful condiment for grilled meats, poultry, or seafood.

Pickled Vegetables:

Ingredients:

- Assorted vegetables (e.g., carrots, cucumbers, bell peppers, cauliflower), sliced or cut into bite-sized pieces
- 1 cup white vinegar
- 1 cup water
- 2 tablespoons sugar
- 1 tablespoon salt
- 2 cloves garlic, peeled and smashed
- Optional: Whole spices like mustard seeds, coriander seeds, black peppercorns, or red pepper flakes for added flavor

Instructions:

1. In a saucepan, combine white vinegar, water, sugar, salt, and smashed garlic cloves.

2. Bring the mixture to a simmer over medium heat, stirring until the sugar and salt dissolve.

3. Remove the pan from heat and let the brine cool to room temperature.

4. Prepare your chosen vegetables by slicing or cutting them into bite-sized pieces.

5. Place the vegetables in a clean, sterilized jar or jars.

6. Optionally, add whole spices like mustard seeds, coriander seeds, black peppercorns, or red pepper flakes to the jar for added flavor.

7. Pour the cooled brine over the vegetables, ensuring they are fully submerged.

8. Seal the jar and refrigerate for at least 24 hours to allow the vegetables to pickle and absorb the flavors.

9. Shake or gently stir the jar occasionally to distribute the flavors evenly.

10. The pickled vegetables can be stored in the refrigerator for several weeks.

Cilantro-Lime Rice:

Ingredients:

- 1 cup long-grain white rice
- 2 cups water or vegetable broth
- 1 tablespoon olive oil
- Juice of 2 limes
- 1/4 cup fresh cilantro, chopped
- Salt to taste

Instructions:

1. Rinse the rice under cold water until the water runs clear to remove excess starch.

2. In a medium saucepan, combine the rinsed rice and water or vegetable broth.

3. Bring the mixture to a boil over medium-high heat, then reduce the heat to low, cover, and simmer for 15-20 minutes or until the rice is cooked and the liquid is absorbed.

4. Once cooked, fluff the rice with a fork to separate the grains.

5. In a small bowl, mix together olive oil, lime juice, chopped fresh cilantro, and a pinch of salt.

6. Pour the cilantro-lime mixture over the cooked rice and gently toss to combine.

7. Taste the rice and adjust the seasoning or add more lime juice if desired.

8. Cover the rice and let it sit for a few minutes to allow the flavors to meld.

9. Serve the cilantro-lime rice as a flavorful side dish to complement your favorite main courses.

Roasted Garlic:

Ingredients:
- Whole garlic bulbs
- Olive oil
- Salt and pepper to taste

Instructions:
1. Preheat your oven to 400°F (200°C).
2. Peel away the loose outer layers of the garlic bulb, leaving the individual cloves intact.
3. Using a sharp knife, trim about 1/4 inch off the top of each garlic bulb, exposing the tops of the cloves.
4. Place the garlic bulbs in a baking dish or on a piece of foil.
5. Drizzle olive oil over the exposed cloves, ensuring they are well-coated.
6. Sprinkle salt and pepper over the garlic bulbs.
7. Cover the garlic bulbs loosely with foil if using a baking dish or wrap them in the foil if placed directly on the oven rack.
8. Roast in the preheated oven for 30-40 minutes or until the cloves are soft and golden brown.
9. Let the roasted garlic cool slightly before handling.
10. Squeeze the garlic cloves out of their skins, and use the roasted garlic in recipes or spread it on bread.

Soy Sauce or Tamari:

Ingredients:
- 1 cup beef or vegetable broth
- 2 tablespoons balsamic vinegar
- 1 tablespoon dark molasses
- 1 teaspoon sesame oil
- 1/4 teaspoon garlic powder
- 1/4 teaspoon ground black pepper

Instructions:
1. In a small saucepan, combine beef or vegetable broth, balsamic vinegar, dark molasses, sesame oil, garlic powder, and black pepper.

2. Bring the mixture to a simmer over medium heat.
3. Reduce heat to low and let it simmer for about 10-15 minutes, allowing the flavors to meld.
4. Taste and adjust the ingredients as needed to achieve a balance of sweetness, saltiness, and umami.
5. Once satisfied with the flavor, let the soy sauce alternative cool before using.

Cranberry Sauce:

Ingredients:

- 1 cup fresh or frozen cranberries
- 1/2 cup granulated sugar
- 1/2 cup water
- Optional: Orange zest or juice, cinnamon, or chopped nuts for added flavor

Instructions:

1. Rinse the cranberries under cold water and remove any stems or blemished berries.
2. In a saucepan, combine cranberries, sugar, and water.
3. If desired, add optional ingredients such as orange zest, a splash of orange juice, a pinch of cinnamon, or chopped nuts for extra flavor.
4. Bring the mixture to a boil over medium-high heat, stirring occasionally.
5. Reduce the heat to low and let it simmer for about 10-15 minutes, or until the cranberries burst and the sauce thickens.
6. Taste the cranberry sauce and adjust the sweetness if needed by adding more sugar.
7. Once the cranberry sauce reaches your desired consistency, remove it from the heat.
8. Let the sauce cool to room temperature before transferring it to a serving dish.
9. Refrigerate the cranberry sauce for at least a couple of hours before serving to enhance the flavors.

CHAPTER 9: SWEET TREATS AND SPECIAL OCCASION RECIPES

Dark Chocolate:

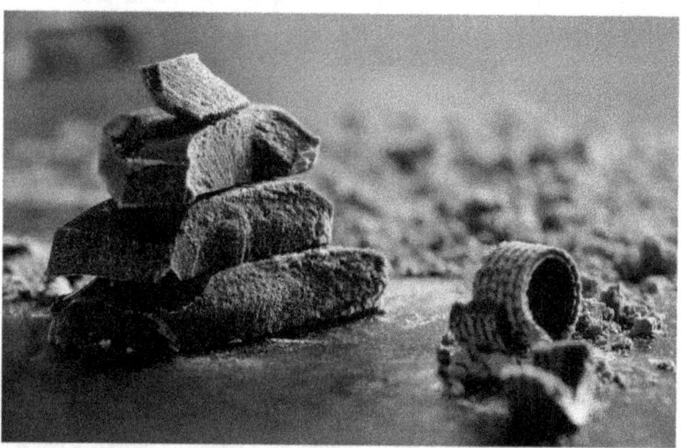

Ingredients:

- 1 cup dark chocolate chips or chopped dark chocolate
- 1 cup nuts of your choice (almonds, cashews, walnuts, etc.)

Instructions:

1. Line a baking sheet with parchment paper.
2. In a heatproof bowl, melt the dark chocolate using a double boiler or microwave in short intervals, stirring in between until smooth.
3. Once melted, remove the chocolate from heat and let it cool slightly.
4. Add nuts to the melted chocolate, stirring until they are well coated.
5. Using a fork or a spoon, scoop out the chocolate-coated nuts one by one, allowing excess chocolate to drip back into the bowl.
6. Place the chocolate-covered nuts on the prepared baking sheet, ensuring they are not touching each other.

7. Let the chocolate-covered nuts set at room temperature or refrigerate for quicker setting.

8. Once set, store the dark chocolate-covered nuts in an airtight container.

Mixed Berries with Almonds:

Ingredients:

- 2 cups mixed berries (strawberries, blueberries, raspberries, blackberries)
- 1/4 cup sliced almonds
- 1-2 tablespoons honey or maple syrup
- Optional: Fresh mint leaves for garnish

Instructions:

1. Wash and prepare the mixed berries as needed. If using strawberries, hull and slice them.

2. In a dry skillet over medium heat, toast the sliced almonds until they become golden brown and fragrant. Be attentive and stir frequently to avoid burning.

3. In a serving bowl, combine the mixed berries and toasted almonds.

4. Drizzle honey or maple syrup over the berries and almonds. Adjust the sweetness to your liking.

5. Gently toss the berries and almonds to coat them evenly with the honey or maple syrup.

6. Let the mixed berries sit for a few minutes to allow the flavors to meld.

7. Optionally, garnish with fresh mint leaves for a burst of freshness.

8. Serve the mixed berries with almonds as a delightful and nutritious dessert, snack, or breakfast topping.

Almond Butter Banana Bites:

Ingredients:

- 2 large bananas, peeled and sliced into rounds
- Almond butter

- Optional toppings: Chia seeds, shredded coconut, sliced almonds, or a drizzle of honey

Instructions:

1. Lay the banana slices on a plate or tray.
2. Spread a small amount of almond butter on each banana slice.
3. Optionally, sprinkle toppings such as chia seeds, shredded coconut, sliced almonds, or drizzle honey over the almond butter.
4. If desired, sandwich two banana slices together with almond butter in the middle to create banana bites.
5. Arrange the almond butter banana bites on a serving plate.
6. Optionally, chill in the refrigerator for a short time to firm up slightly.
7. Serve and enjoy these simple and nutritious almond butter banana bites as a healthy snack or dessert.

Baked Apples:

Ingredients:

- 4 large apples (such as Granny Smith or Honeycrisp)
- 1/4 cup brown sugar
- 1 teaspoon ground cinnamon
- 1/4 teaspoon ground nutmeg
- 2 tablespoons unsalted butter, cut into small pieces
- 1/2 cup water or apple juice
- Optional: Chopped nuts, raisins, or a drizzle of honey for topping

Instructions:

1. Preheat your oven to 375°F (190°C).
2. Wash and core the apples, leaving the bottoms intact.
3. In a small bowl, mix together brown sugar, ground cinnamon, and ground nutmeg.
4. Place the cored apples in a baking dish.
5. Stuff each apple with the brown sugar mixture, dividing it evenly among them.

6. Place small pieces of butter on top of the brown sugar mixture in each apple.

7. Pour water or apple juice into the bottom of the baking dish to prevent the apples from drying out during baking.

8. Optionally, sprinkle chopped nuts or raisins over the top of the apples.

9. Cover the baking dish with foil and bake in the preheated oven for 25-30 minutes or until the apples are tender.

10. Remove the foil and bake for an additional 5-10 minutes to allow the tops to caramelize.

11. Once baked, let the apples cool for a few minutes before serving.

12. Optionally, drizzle honey over the baked apples before serving.

Chia Pudding with Berries:

Ingredients:

- 1/4 cup chia seeds
- 1 cup milk (dairy or plant-based)
- 1 tablespoon maple syrup or honey (adjust to taste)
- 1/2 teaspoon vanilla extract
- Mixed berries (strawberries, blueberries, raspberries) for topping
- Optional: Sliced almonds, shredded coconut, or mint leaves for garnish

Instructions:

1. In a bowl, combine chia seeds, milk, maple syrup (or honey), and vanilla extract.

2. Whisk the mixture thoroughly to ensure the chia seeds are evenly distributed.

3. Let the chia pudding mixture sit for about 5 minutes, then whisk again to prevent clumping.

4. Cover the bowl and refrigerate the chia pudding for at least 2 hours or overnight to allow it to thicken.

5. After the pudding has set, give it a good stir to achieve a creamy consistency.

6. Spoon the chia pudding into serving glasses or bowls.

7. Top the chia pudding with mixed berries.

8. Optionally, garnish with sliced almonds, shredded coconut, or mint leaves for added texture and flavor.

9. Serve the chia pudding with berries chilled.

Coconut Macaroons:

Ingredients:

- 3 cups shredded coconut (unsweetened)
- 3/4 cup sweetened condensed milk
- 1 teaspoon vanilla extract
- 2 large egg whites
- 1/4 teaspoon salt
- Optional: Dark chocolate for drizzling or dipping (melted)

Instructions:

1. Preheat your oven to 325°F (163°C). Line a baking sheet with parchment paper.

2. In a large bowl, combine shredded coconut, sweetened condensed milk, and vanilla extract. Mix well.

3. In a separate bowl, beat the egg whites with salt until stiff peaks form.

4. Gently fold the beaten egg whites into the coconut mixture until evenly combined.

5. Using a spoon or cookie scoop, drop mounds of the coconut mixture onto the prepared baking sheet, leaving some space between each.

6. Bake in the preheated oven for approximately 15-20 minutes or until the edges are golden brown.

7. Allow the coconut macaroons to cool on the baking sheet for a few minutes before transferring them to a wire rack to cool completely.

8. Optionally, melt dark chocolate and drizzle or dip the cooled macaroons for added flavor.

9. Let the chocolate set before serving.

Frozen Yogurt:

Ingredients:

- 3 cups Greek yogurt (full-fat for creamier texture)
- 1/2 cup honey or maple syrup (adjust to taste)
- 1 teaspoon vanilla extract
- 2 cups frozen mixed berries (or fruit of your choice)
- Optional: Lemon zest or juice for a citrusy kick

Instructions:

1. In a blender or food processor, combine Greek yogurt, honey or maple syrup, and vanilla extract.
2. Blend the mixture until smooth and well combined.
3. Add frozen mixed berries to the blender. If the berries are too large, you may want to chop them before adding.
4. Blend again until the frozen berries are fully incorporated, and the mixture has a smooth and creamy consistency.
5. Taste the frozen yogurt base and adjust the sweetness if needed.
6. If desired, add a bit of lemon zest or juice for a citrusy flavor. Blend once more to combine.
7. Transfer the frozen yogurt mixture to a freezer-safe container, spreading it evenly.
8. Cover the container and freeze for at least 4-6 hours or until the frozen yogurt is firm.
9. Before serving, let the frozen yogurt sit at room temperature for a few minutes to soften slightly for easier scooping.
10. Scoop the frozen yogurt into bowls or cones and enjoy!

Pumpkin Custard:

Ingredients:

- 1 can (15 ounces) pumpkin puree
- 3 large eggs

- 1/2 cup brown sugar, packed
- 1 teaspoon ground cinnamon
- 1/2 teaspoon ground ginger
- 1/4 teaspoon ground nutmeg
- 1/4 teaspoon salt
- 1 teaspoon vanilla extract
- 1 cup whole milk or coconut milk (for a dairy-free option)
- Whipped cream and ground cinnamon for garnish (optional)

Instructions:

1. Preheat your oven to 325°F (163°C). Grease individual ramekins or a baking dish.
2. In a large bowl, whisk together pumpkin puree, eggs, brown sugar, cinnamon, ginger, nutmeg, salt, and vanilla extract until well combined.
3. Gradually add the milk to the pumpkin mixture, whisking continuously until smooth.
4. Pour the pumpkin custard mixture into the prepared ramekins or baking dish.
5. Place the ramekins or baking dish in a larger baking pan. Fill the larger pan with hot water until it reaches halfway up the sides of the ramekins or baking dish. This creates a water bath for even baking.
6. Bake in the preheated oven for approximately 40-45 minutes or until the custard is set around the edges but slightly jiggly in the center.
7. Carefully remove the pumpkin custard from the water bath and let it cool to room temperature.
8. Once cooled, cover and refrigerate for at least 2 hours or overnight to allow the custard to set completely.
9. Serve the pumpkin custard chilled, optionally topped with whipped cream and a sprinkle of ground cinnamon.

Date and Nut Bars:

Ingredients:

- 1 cup dates, pitted and chopped
- 1 cup nuts (such as almonds, walnuts, or a mix), chopped
- 1 cup old-fashioned oats
- 1/4 cup honey or maple syrup
- 2 tablespoons nut butter (almond butter, peanut butter, etc.)
- 1/4 cup shredded coconut (optional)
- 1/2 teaspoon vanilla extract
- Pinch of salt

Instructions:

1. In a food processor, combine dates, nuts, oats, honey or maple syrup, nut butter, shredded coconut (if using), vanilla extract, and a pinch of salt.
2. Process the mixture until it forms a sticky and cohesive dough.
3. Line a square baking dish with parchment paper, leaving some overhang for easy removal.
4. Transfer the mixture to the baking dish and press it down firmly and evenly.
5. Place the baking dish in the refrigerator for at least 1-2 hours to allow the mixture to set.
6. Once set, use the parchment paper overhang to lift the date and nut slab from the baking dish.
7. Cut the slab into bars or squares of your desired size.
8. Store the date and nut bars in an airtight container in the refrigerator for freshness.

Peach Sorbet:

Ingredients:

- 4 cups ripe peaches, peeled, pitted, and sliced
- 1/2 cup granulated sugar (adjust based on sweetness of peaches)
- 1 tablespoon lemon juice
- 1/2 cup water
- Optional: Mint leaves for garnish

Instructions:

1. In a blender or food processor, combine sliced peaches, granulated sugar, lemon juice, and water.
2. Blend the mixture until smooth and well combined.
3. Taste the peach mixture and adjust the sweetness if needed by adding more sugar.
4. Strain the peach mixture through a fine-mesh sieve to remove any remaining solids. This step is optional, depending on your preference for texture.
5. Pour the strained peach puree into a shallow dish or pan.
6. Place the dish in the freezer and let it freeze for about 1-2 hours.
7. After the initial freeze, use a fork to scrape and fluff the partially frozen sorbet.
8. Repeat the scraping process every 30 minutes for the next 2-3 hours or until the sorbet reaches a smooth and scoopable consistency.
9. Once the peach sorbet is fully frozen and has a desired texture, transfer it to a sealed container and store it in the freezer.
10. Before serving, let the sorbet sit at room temperature for a few minutes to soften slightly.
11. Scoop the peach sorbet into bowls or cones.
12. Optionally, garnish with fresh mint leaves.

Banana Ice Cream:

Ingredients:

- 4 ripe bananas, peeled, sliced, and frozen
- 1 teaspoon vanilla extract (optional)
- Optional toppings: Nuts, chocolate chips, honey, or sliced fruit

Instructions:

1. Slice ripe bananas and place the slices in a single layer on a parchment paper-lined tray or plate.
2. Freeze the banana slices for at least 2 hours or until solid.
3. Transfer the frozen banana slices to a blender or food processor.

4. Blend the frozen banana slices until they resemble a creamy, smooth consistency. This may take a few minutes, and you may need to stop and scrape down the sides of the blender or food processor.

5. Optionally, add vanilla extract to the blended banana for extra flavor. Blend again to incorporate.

6. Taste the banana ice cream and adjust the sweetness or flavor if desired.

7. Serve the banana ice cream immediately for a soft-serve consistency, or transfer it to a container and freeze for an additional 1-2 hours for a firmer texture.

8. Before serving, let the banana ice cream soften for a few minutes at room temperature.

9. Optionally, top with nuts, chocolate chips, honey, or sliced fruit before serving.

Yogurt Parfait:

Ingredients:

- 2 cups Greek yogurt (or your favorite yogurt)
- 1 cup granola
- 1 cup mixed berries (strawberries, blueberries, raspberries)
- Honey for drizzling
- Optional: Chia seeds, sliced almonds, or shredded coconut for added texture

Instructions:

1. In serving glasses or bowls, layer the bottom with a spoonful of Greek yogurt.

2. Add a layer of granola on top of the yogurt.

3. Place a layer of mixed berries over the granola.

4. Drizzle honey over the berries.

5. Repeat the layers until you reach the top of the glass or bowl.

6. Optionally, sprinkle chia seeds, sliced almonds, or shredded coconut between the layers for added texture.

7. Finish with a final drizzle of honey on top.

8. Repeat the layering process for each parfait.

9. Serve the yogurt parfaits immediately as a delicious and nutritious breakfast or snack.

Special Occasion Recipes:

Grilled Steak with Garlic Butter:

Ingredients:

- 2 boneless ribeye or sirloin steaks (about 1 inch thick)
- Salt and black pepper to season
- 2 tablespoons olive oil
- 4 cloves garlic, minced
- 4 tablespoons unsalted butter
- Fresh parsley, chopped (for garnish)

Instructions:

1. Preheat your grill to medium-high heat.
2. Season the steaks generously with salt and black pepper on both sides.
3. Drizzle olive oil over the steaks and rub it in to coat them evenly.
4. Place the steaks on the preheated grill and cook to your desired doneness, turning once. Cooking times will vary based on the thickness of the steaks and your grill's heat.
5. While the steaks are cooking, prepare the garlic butter. In a small saucepan, melt the butter over medium heat.
6. Add minced garlic to the melted butter and sauté for 1-2 minutes until the garlic becomes fragrant. Be careful not to brown the garlic too much.
7. Once the steaks are cooked to your liking, transfer them to a plate.
8. Pour the garlic butter over the grilled steaks, ensuring they are well coated.
9. Let the steaks rest for a few minutes before slicing.
10. Garnish with chopped fresh parsley and serve.

Roast Turkey with Cranberry Sauce:

Ingredients:

- 1 whole turkey (12-14 pounds), thawed if frozen
- Salt and black pepper for seasoning
- 1 cup unsalted butter, melted
- 1 tablespoon dried thyme
- 1 tablespoon dried rosemary
- 1 tablespoon dried sage
- 1 cup chicken or turkey broth

For the Cranberry Sauce:

- 1 cup fresh or frozen cranberries
- 1/2 cup orange juice
- 1/2 cup granulated sugar
- Zest of 1 orange

Instructions:

1. Preparing the Turkey:

- Preheat your oven to 325°F (163°C).
- Remove the giblets and neck from the turkey cavity.
- Rinse the turkey inside and out, pat it dry with paper towels.
- Season the turkey cavity with salt and pepper.
- In a small bowl, mix melted butter, dried thyme, rosemary, and sage.
- Place the turkey on a rack in a roasting pan.
- Brush the turkey with the herb-infused melted butter, and season generously with salt and pepper.
- Tent the turkey with aluminum foil.

2. Roasting the Turkey:

- Roast the turkey in the preheated oven, allowing about 15 minutes per pound.
- Baste the turkey with the pan juices and melted butter every 30 minutes.
- Remove the foil during the last hour of roasting to allow the skin to brown.

3. Checking Doneness:

  - Use a meat thermometer to ensure the turkey's internal temperature reaches 165°F (74°C) in the thickest part of the thigh without touching the bone.

4. Resting the Turkey:

  - Once done, let the turkey rest for at least 20-30 minutes before carving.

5. Making Cranberry Sauce:

  - While the turkey is roasting, combine cranberries, orange juice, sugar, and orange zest in a saucepan.
  - Bring the mixture to a boil, then reduce heat and simmer until the cranberries burst and the sauce thickens.

6. Serving:

  - Carve the turkey and arrange the slices on a serving platter.
  - Serve with the homemade cranberry sauce on the side.

Lobster Tail with Garlic Butter:

Ingredients:

  - 4 lobster tails
  - Salt and black pepper to season
  - 1/2 cup unsalted butter
  - 4 cloves garlic, minced
  - 1 tablespoon fresh parsley, chopped
  - 1 tablespoon fresh lemon juice
  - Lemon wedges for serving

Instructions:

1. Preparing the Lobster Tails:

  - Thaw lobster tails if frozen by placing them in the refrigerator overnight.
  - Use kitchen shears to cut along the top of the lobster shell, stopping at the base of the tail. Gently lift the meat through the slit, keeping it attached at the base.

2. Seasoning:

- Season the lobster meat with salt and black pepper.

3. Broiling:
- Preheat your oven broiler.
- Place the lobster tails on a baking sheet, shell side down.
- Broil for about 5-7 minutes or until the lobster meat is opaque and slightly browned.

4. Preparing Garlic Butter:
- While the lobster is broiling, melt butter in a saucepan over medium heat.
- Add minced garlic and sauté for 1-2 minutes until fragrant.
- Stir in chopped parsley and lemon juice. Remove from heat.

5. Serving:
- Once the lobster tails are done, brush them generously with the garlic butter mixture.
- Optionally, pour a bit of the garlic butter onto the serving plate.
- Serve lobster tails with lemon wedges on the side.

Rack of Lamb:

Ingredients:
- 2 racks of lamb (8 ribs each)
- 4 cloves garlic, minced
- 2 tablespoons fresh rosemary, chopped
- 2 tablespoons Dijon mustard
- Salt and black pepper to taste
- 2 tablespoons olive oil

Instructions:
1. Preheat Oven: Preheat your oven to 400°F (200°C).
2. Prepare the Lamb: Trim excess fat from the racks of lamb. Season with salt and black pepper.

3. Create Herb Rub: In a small bowl, mix minced garlic, chopped rosemary, Dijon mustard, and olive oil to form a paste.

4. Coat Lamb: Rub the lamb racks with the herb paste, ensuring an even coating.

5. Sear the Lamb: In a hot skillet, sear the lamb racks on all sides until browned. This step adds flavor and helps seal in juices.

6. Roasting: Place the seared racks on a roasting pan, bones facing down. Roast in the preheated oven for about 20-25 minutes for medium-rare. Adjust time for desired doneness.

7. Resting: Allow the lamb to rest for 10 minutes before slicing. This ensures the juices redistribute, keeping the meat moist.

8. Serving: Slice between the ribs and serve the succulent roasted rack of lamb. Optionally, garnish with additional fresh herbs.

Stuffed Bell Peppers:

Ingredients:

- 4 large bell peppers (any color)
- 1 lb (450g) ground beef or turkey
- 1 cup cooked rice
- 1 onion, finely chopped
- 2 cloves garlic, minced
- 1 can (14 oz) diced tomatoes, drained
- 1 cup shredded cheese (cheddar, mozzarella, or your choice)
- 1 teaspoon dried oregano
- 1 teaspoon ground cumin
- Salt and black pepper to taste
- Olive oil for cooking

Instructions:

1. Preheat Oven: Preheat your oven to 375°F (190°C).

2. Prepare Bell Peppers: Cut the tops off the bell peppers and remove seeds and membranes. Lightly brush the exterior with olive oil.

3. Sauté Onion and Garlic: In a pan over medium heat, sauté chopped onion and minced garlic until softened.

4. Cook Ground Meat: Add ground beef or turkey to the pan and cook until browned. Drain excess fat.

5. Combine Ingredients: In a large bowl, mix cooked meat, cooked rice, diced tomatoes, half of the shredded cheese, oregano, cumin, salt, and black pepper.

6. Stuff Peppers: Spoon the mixture into the hollowed-out bell peppers. Top each with the remaining shredded cheese.

7. Bake: Place the stuffed peppers in a baking dish and bake in the preheated oven for about 25-30 minutes or until peppers are tender.

8. Serve: Once cooked, remove from the oven and let them cool slightly before serving.

Salmon en Papillote:

Ingredients:

- 4 salmon fillets (6 oz each)
- 4 sheets of parchment paper (about 12x16 inches)
- 1 lemon, thinly sliced
- 4 sprigs of fresh dill
- 2 tablespoons olive oil
- Salt and black pepper to taste
- 4 tablespoons dry white wine or chicken broth
- Optional: Sliced vegetables like asparagus or cherry tomatoes

Instructions:

1. Preheat Oven: Preheat your oven to 400°F (200°C).

2. Prepare Parchment Packets: Fold each sheet of parchment paper in half and cut into a heart shape. Open the heart-shaped paper and place a salmon fillet on one side.

3. Season Salmon: Drizzle each fillet with olive oil and season with salt and black pepper. Place lemon slices on top of each fillet, add a sprig of dill, and any optional vegetables.

4. Fold and Seal Packets: Fold the parchment paper over the salmon, creating a half-moon shape. Starting at the top of the heart, make small overlapping folds to seal the edges, creating a sealed packet.

5. Add Liquid: Before sealing completely, pour 1 tablespoon of white wine or chicken broth into each packet.

6. Bake: Place the sealed packets on a baking sheet and bake in the preheated oven for about 12-15 minutes, depending on the thickness of the salmon. The packets will puff up as they cook.

7. Serve: Carefully open the packets (watch out for steam) and transfer the salmon, along with the lemon and juices, to a plate.

8. Garnish: Garnish with additional fresh dill and serve the salmon en papillote directly in the parchment paper for an elegant presentation.

Vegetable and Shrimp Stir-Fry:

Ingredients:
- 1 lb (450g) large shrimp, peeled and deveined
- 4 cups mixed vegetables (broccoli florets, bell peppers, snap peas, carrots, etc.), sliced
- 3 cloves garlic, minced
- 1 tablespoon fresh ginger, grated
- 3 tablespoons soy sauce
- 1 tablespoon oyster sauce
- 1 tablespoon hoisin sauce

- 1 tablespoon sesame oil
- 2 tablespoons vegetable oil (for cooking)
- 2 green onions, sliced (for garnish)
- Cooked rice or noodles for serving

Instructions:

1. Prepare Shrimp: Pat the shrimp dry with paper towels. Season with salt and black pepper.
2. Mix Sauce: In a small bowl, whisk together soy sauce, oyster sauce, hoisin sauce, and sesame oil. Set aside.
3. Heat Pan: Heat vegetable oil in a wok or large skillet over medium-high heat.
4. Cook Shrimp: Add shrimp to the hot pan and cook for 2-3 minutes on each side until they turn pink and opaque. Remove shrimp from the pan and set aside.
5. Sauté Vegetables: In the same pan, add a bit more oil if needed. Sauté garlic and ginger until fragrant. Add the sliced vegetables and stir-fry for 3-5 minutes until they are crisp-tender.
6. Combine Ingredients: Return the cooked shrimp to the pan. Pour the sauce over the shrimp and vegetables. Toss everything together until well-coated and heated through.
7. Garnish: Sprinkle sliced green onions over the stir-fry for a fresh finish.
8. Serve: Serve the vegetable and shrimp stir-fry over cooked rice or noodles.

Grilled Portobello Mushrooms:

Ingredients:

- 4 large Portobello mushrooms
- 3 tablespoons balsamic vinegar
- 2 tablespoons olive oil
- 2 cloves garlic, minced
- 1 teaspoon dried thyme
- Salt and black pepper to taste

- Optional: Fresh parsley for garnish

Instructions:

1. Clean Mushrooms: Wipe the Portobello mushrooms with a damp cloth to remove any dirt. Remove the stems and gently scrape out the gills using a spoon.
2. Prepare Marinade: In a small bowl, whisk together balsamic vinegar, olive oil, minced garlic, dried thyme, salt, and black pepper.
3. Marinate Mushrooms: Place the cleaned mushrooms in a shallow dish or a large zip-top bag. Pour the marinade over the mushrooms, ensuring they are well-coated. Allow them to marinate for at least 15-30 minutes.
4. Preheat Grill: Preheat your grill to medium-high heat.
5. Grill Mushrooms: Place the marinated Portobello mushrooms on the preheated grill, gill side down. Grill for about 4-5 minutes per side or until they are tender and have grill marks.
6. Baste with Marinade: Occasionally brush the mushrooms with the marinade during grilling for added flavor.
7. Serve: Once grilled, transfer the mushrooms to a serving plate. Optionally, garnish with fresh parsley.
8. Enjoy: Serve the Grilled Portobello Mushrooms as a side dish, on a salad, or as a meaty topping for burgers.

Chicken Marsala:

Ingredients:

- 4 boneless, skinless chicken breasts
- 1/2 cup all-purpose flour, for dredging
- Salt and black pepper to taste
- 4 tablespoons olive oil
- 8 oz (225g) mushrooms, sliced
- 3/4 cup Marsala wine
- 1/2 cup chicken broth

- 2 tablespoons unsalted butter
- 2 tablespoons fresh parsley, chopped (for garnish)

Instructions:

1. Prepare Chicken: Season chicken breasts with salt and black pepper. Dredge each piece in flour, shaking off excess.
2. Sear Chicken: In a large skillet, heat olive oil over medium-high heat. Add chicken breasts and cook for about 4-5 minutes per side or until golden brown and cooked through. Remove chicken from the pan and set aside.
3. Sauté Mushrooms: In the same skillet, add a bit more oil if needed. Sauté the sliced mushrooms until they release their juices and become golden brown.
4. Deglaze with Marsala Wine: Pour Marsala wine into the skillet, scraping the brown bits from the bottom of the pan. Allow the wine to reduce by half.
5. Add Chicken Broth: Pour in chicken broth and simmer for a few minutes to combine flavors.
6. Return Chicken to Pan: Return the cooked chicken breasts to the skillet, simmering for an additional 5 minutes to let the flavors meld.
7. Finish with Butter: Stir in butter to create a rich, silky sauce. Adjust seasoning with salt and black pepper if needed.
8. Garnish and Serve: Sprinkle chopped fresh parsley over the Chicken Marsala just before serving. Serve the chicken with the Marsala sauce poured over the top.

Vegetable Lasagna:

Ingredients:

- 9 lasagna noodles, cooked according to package instructions
- 2 cups ricotta cheese
- 1 egg
- 1 cup grated Parmesan cheese
- 3 cups shredded mozzarella cheese
- 1 zucchini, thinly sliced

- 1 yellow squash, thinly sliced
- 1 bell pepper, diced
- 1 cup sliced mushrooms
- 1 onion, finely chopped
- 3 cloves garlic, minced
- 1 can (28 oz) crushed tomatoes
- 2 tablespoons tomato paste
- 2 teaspoons dried oregano
- 1 teaspoon dried basil
- Salt and black pepper to taste
- Olive oil for cooking

Instructions:

1. Preheat Oven: Preheat your oven to 375°F (190°C).
2. Prepare Vegetables: In a pan, sauté onions and garlic in olive oil until softened. Add diced bell pepper, sliced zucchini, yellow squash, and mushrooms. Cook until the vegetables are tender. Season with salt and black pepper.
3. Prepare Sauce: Stir in crushed tomatoes, tomato paste, dried oregano, and dried basil into the vegetable mixture. Simmer for 10-15 minutes, allowing the flavors to meld. Adjust seasoning if needed.
4. Prepare Ricotta Mixture: In a bowl, mix ricotta cheese, egg, and grated Parmesan cheese until well combined.
5. Assemble Lasagna: In a baking dish, spread a thin layer of the tomato sauce mixture. Place a layer of cooked lasagna noodles on top. Spread half of the ricotta mixture over the noodles. Add a layer of the sautéed vegetables. Sprinkle with mozzarella cheese. Repeat the layers, finishing with a layer of sauce and mozzarella cheese on top.
6. Bake: Cover the baking dish with foil and bake in the preheated oven for 25 minutes. Remove the foil and bake for an additional 10-15 minutes or until the cheese is bubbly and golden.

7. Rest Before Serving: Allow the vegetable lasagna to rest for 10 minutes before slicing.

8. Serve: Serve warm, and enjoy your delicious and hearty Vegetable Lasagna!

Wild Rice Stuffed Acorn Squash:

Ingredients:

- 2 acorn squash, halved and seeds removed
- 1 cup wild rice, cooked according to package instructions
- 1 cup mushrooms, diced
- 1/2 cup celery, finely chopped
- 1/2 cup onion, finely chopped
- 2 cloves garlic, minced
- 1/2 cup dried cranberries
- 1/2 cup pecans, chopped
- 2 tablespoons olive oil
- 1 teaspoon dried thyme
- Salt and black pepper to taste
- Fresh parsley for garnish

Instructions:

1. Preheat Oven: Preheat your oven to 375°F (190°C).

2. Prepare Acorn Squash: Place acorn squash halves on a baking sheet, cut side up. Brush the cut sides with olive oil, sprinkle with salt and black pepper. Roast in the preheated oven for 30-40 minutes or until tender.

3. Sauté Vegetables: In a pan, heat olive oil over medium heat. Add onions, garlic, mushrooms, and celery. Sauté until the vegetables are softened.

4. Combine Ingredients: In a large bowl, mix the cooked wild rice, sautéed vegetables, dried cranberries, chopped pecans, and dried thyme. Season with salt and black pepper to taste.

5. Stuff Acorn Squash: Once the acorn squash halves are tender, fill each half with the wild rice mixture.

6. Bake Again: Return the stuffed acorn squash to the oven and bake for an additional 15-20 minutes or until the filling is heated through and the tops are golden.

7. Garnish and Serve: Sprinkle fresh parsley over the stuffed acorn squash before serving.

8. Enjoy: Serve warm and enjoy the delightful combination of flavors and textures in this Wild Rice Stuffed Acorn Squash!

Tofu and Vegetable Skewers:

Ingredients:

- 14 oz (400g) extra-firm tofu, pressed and cubed
- 2 bell peppers (assorted colors), cut into chunks
- 1 zucchini, sliced into rounds
- 1 red onion, cut into wedges
- Cherry tomatoes
- 2 tablespoons soy sauce
- 2 tablespoons olive oil
- 1 tablespoon maple syrup or honey
- 1 teaspoon ground cumin
- 1 teaspoon smoked paprika
- 1 teaspoon garlic powder
- Salt and black pepper to taste
- Wooden skewers, soaked in water for at least 30 minutes

Instructions:

1. Prepare Tofu: Press the tofu to remove excess water, then cut it into cubes.

2. Marinate Tofu: In a bowl, whisk together soy sauce, olive oil, maple syrup or honey, ground cumin, smoked paprika, garlic powder, salt, and black pepper. Toss the tofu cubes in the marinade and let it marinate for at least 15-30 minutes.

3. Prepare Vegetables: While the tofu is marinating, prepare the vegetables by cutting them into chunks or slices.

4. Assemble Skewers: Thread the marinated tofu cubes and assorted vegetables onto the soaked wooden skewers, alternating between tofu and vegetables.

5. Grill or Oven-Bake:
   - Grill: Preheat your grill to medium-high heat. Grill the skewers for about 10-15 minutes, turning occasionally until the tofu is golden brown and the vegetables are tender.
   - Oven: Preheat your oven to 400°F (200°C). Place the skewers on a baking sheet and bake for 20-25 minutes, turning halfway through.

6. Baste with Marinade: During grilling or baking, baste the skewers with any remaining marinade for added flavor.

7. Serve: Once cooked, remove from the grill or oven. Serve the tofu and vegetable skewers hot, and optionally, garnish with fresh herbs.

CHAPTER 10: SALAD AND BEVERAGES

Salads:

Grilled Chicken Caesar Salad:

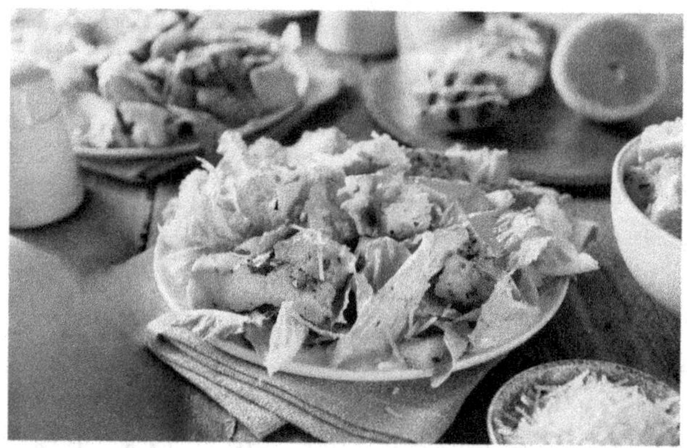

Ingredients:

- 2 boneless, skinless chicken breasts
- Salt and black pepper to taste
- 2 tablespoons olive oil
- 1 teaspoon garlic powder
- 1 teaspoon dried oregano
- 1 head romaine lettuce, washed and chopped
- 1 cup cherry tomatoes, halved
- 1/2 cup croutons
- 1/2 cup grated Parmesan cheese

Caesar Dressing:

- 1/2 cup mayonnaise
- 2 tablespoons grated Parmesan cheese

- 2 tablespoons lemon juice
- 1 tablespoon Dijon mustard
- 1 teaspoon Worcestershire sauce
- 2 cloves garlic, minced
- Salt and black pepper to taste

Instructions:

1. Preheat the grill to medium-high heat.
2. Season chicken breasts with salt, black pepper, garlic powder, and dried oregano. Drizzle olive oil over the chicken.
3. Grill the chicken for about 6-8 minutes per side, or until fully cooked and grill marks appear. Allow the chicken to rest for a few minutes before slicing it into strips.
4. In a bowl, whisk together all the Caesar dressing ingredients until well combined. Adjust salt and pepper to taste.
5. In a large salad bowl, combine chopped romaine lettuce, cherry tomatoes, croutons, and grilled chicken strips.
6. Pour the Caesar dressing over the salad and toss until everything is evenly coated.
7. Sprinkle grated Parmesan cheese over the top and serve immediately.

Spinach and Walnut Salad:

Ingredients:

- 6 cups fresh baby spinach, washed and dried
- 1 cup cherry tomatoes, halved
- 1/2 cup red onion, thinly sliced
- 1/2 cup feta cheese, crumbled
- 1/2 cup walnuts, toasted
- 2 tablespoons balsamic vinegar
- 3 tablespoons extra-virgin olive oil
- 1 tablespoon honey
- Salt and black pepper to taste

Instructions:

1. In a large salad bowl, combine the fresh baby spinach, cherry tomatoes, sliced red onion, crumbled feta cheese, and toasted walnuts.
2. In a small bowl, whisk together balsamic vinegar, extra-virgin olive oil, honey, salt, and black pepper to create the dressing.
3. Drizzle the dressing over the salad ingredients.
4. Toss the salad gently until the dressing evenly coats the spinach and other ingredients.
5. Serve immediately, ensuring the salad is well-mixed, or you can refrigerate it briefly if you prefer a chilled salad.
6. Optionally, garnish with additional feta cheese and walnuts before serving.

Greek Salad:

Ingredients:

- 4 cups cucumber, diced
- 4 cups tomatoes, diced
- 1 cup red onion, thinly sliced
- 1 cup Kalamata olives, pitted
- 1 cup feta cheese, crumbled
- 1/2 cup fresh parsley, chopped
- 1/4 cup extra-virgin olive oil
- 2 tablespoons red wine vinegar
- 1 teaspoon dried oregano
- Salt and black pepper to taste

Instructions:

1. In a large salad bowl, combine diced cucumber, diced tomatoes, thinly sliced red onion, Kalamata olives, crumbled feta cheese, and chopped fresh parsley.
2. In a small bowl, whisk together extra-virgin olive oil, red wine vinegar, dried oregano, salt, and black pepper to create the dressing.
3. Drizzle the dressing over the salad ingredients.
4. Toss the salad gently until the dressing evenly coats the vegetables and feta.
5. Allow the salad to marinate for a few minutes to enhance the flavors.

6. Serve chilled and enjoy your authentic Greek Salad!

Tuna Salad:

Ingredients:

- 2 cans (5 oz each) tuna, drained
- 1/2 cup celery, finely chopped
- 1/4 cup red onion, finely diced
- 1/4 cup dill pickles, finely chopped
- 1/4 cup mayonnaise
- 1 tablespoon Dijon mustard
- 1 tablespoon fresh lemon juice
- Salt and black pepper to taste
- 4 cups mixed salad greens (optional for serving)

Instructions:

1. In a large mixing bowl, combine drained tuna, chopped celery, diced red onion, and chopped dill pickles.
2. In a separate small bowl, whisk together mayonnaise, Dijon mustard, fresh lemon juice, salt, and black pepper.
3. Pour the dressing over the tuna mixture and gently toss until all ingredients are well coated.
4. Taste and adjust seasoning if needed.
5. Refrigerate the tuna salad for at least 30 minutes to allow flavors to meld.
6. Serve the tuna salad on a bed of mixed salad greens, in a sandwich, or with crackers.
7. Garnish with additional fresh herbs or lemon wedges if desired.

Quinoa and Black Bean Salad:

Ingredients:

- 1 cup quinoa, rinsed and cooked according to package instructions

- 1 can (15 oz) black beans, drained and rinsed
- 1 cup corn kernels (fresh, frozen, or canned)
- 1 red bell pepper, diced
- 1/2 cup red onion, finely chopped
- 1/4 cup fresh cilantro, chopped
- 1 avocado, diced (optional)
- Juice of 2 limes
- 3 tablespoons extra-virgin olive oil
- 1 teaspoon ground cumin
- Salt and black pepper to taste

Instructions:

1. Cook quinoa according to package instructions, then let it cool to room temperature.
2. In a large mixing bowl, combine cooked quinoa, black beans, corn kernels, diced red bell pepper, finely chopped red onion, and chopped fresh cilantro.
3. In a small bowl, whisk together lime juice, extra-virgin olive oil, ground cumin, salt, and black pepper to create the dressing.
4. Pour the dressing over the quinoa and black bean mixture.
5. Toss the salad gently until all ingredients are well coated.
6. Gently fold in diced avocado if using.
7. Refrigerate the salad for at least 30 minutes before serving to enhance flavors.
8. Serve chilled as a refreshing side dish or a light meal.

Asian-Inspired Chicken Salad:

Ingredients:

- 2 boneless, skinless chicken breasts
- Salt and black pepper to taste
- 2 tablespoons soy sauce
- 1 tablespoon sesame oil
- 1 tablespoon rice vinegar

- 1 tablespoon honey
- 1 teaspoon grated ginger
- 1 clove garlic, minced
- 4 cups mixed salad greens
- 1 cup shredded cabbage
- 1 cup shredded carrots
- 1/2 cup sliced cucumber
- 1/4 cup chopped green onions
- 1/4 cup chopped cilantro
- 1/4 cup chopped peanuts or sesame seeds for garnish

Instructions:

1. Season chicken breasts with salt and black pepper.
2. In a bowl, whisk together soy sauce, sesame oil, rice vinegar, honey, grated ginger, and minced garlic to create the marinade.
3. Place chicken breasts in a zip-top bag or shallow dish and pour half of the marinade over them. Allow the chicken to marinate for at least 15-20 minutes.
4. Preheat a grill or grill pan over medium-high heat. Grill the chicken for about 6-8 minutes per side, or until fully cooked. Allow the chicken to rest for a few minutes before slicing it into strips.
5. In a large salad bowl, combine mixed salad greens, shredded cabbage, shredded carrots, sliced cucumber, chopped green onions, and chopped cilantro.
6. Add the sliced grilled chicken on top of the salad.
7. Drizzle the remaining marinade over the salad as a dressing.
8. Garnish with chopped peanuts or sesame seeds.
9. Toss the salad gently to combine all the ingredients.
10. Serve immediately and enjoy your flavorful Asian-Inspired Chicken Salad!

Kale and Cranberry Salad:

Ingredients:

- 6 cups kale, stems removed and leaves thinly sliced
- 1/2 cup dried cranberries
- 1/2 cup feta cheese, crumbled
- 1/4 cup pumpkin seeds (pepitas), toasted
- 1/4 cup red onion, thinly sliced
- 2 tablespoons extra-virgin olive oil

- 2 tablespoons balsamic vinegar
- 1 tablespoon honey
- 1 teaspoon Dijon mustard
- Salt and black pepper to taste

Instructions:

1. In a large mixing bowl, combine thinly sliced kale, dried cranberries, crumbled feta cheese, toasted pumpkin seeds, and thinly sliced red onion.
2. In a small bowl, whisk together extra-virgin olive oil, balsamic vinegar, honey, Dijon mustard, salt, and black pepper to create the dressing.
3. Pour the dressing over the kale mixture.
4. Using your hands, gently massage the dressing into the kale for a few minutes. This helps to soften the kale and infuse it with flavor.
5. Let the salad sit for about 10 minutes to allow the flavors to meld.
6. Toss the salad gently once more before serving.
7. Optionally, garnish with additional feta cheese and pumpkin seeds.
8. Serve immediately as a side dish or a light, nutritious meal.

Mango Avocado Salad:

Ingredients:

- 2 ripe mangos, peeled, pitted, and diced
- 2 ripe avocados, peeled, pitted, and diced
- 1 cup cherry tomatoes, halved
- 1/4 cup red onion, finely chopped
- 1/4 cup fresh cilantro, chopped
- Juice of 2 limes
- 2 tablespoons extra-virgin olive oil
- Salt and black pepper to taste
- Optional: 1 jalapeño, seeded and finely chopped for some heat

Instructions:

1. In a large salad bowl, combine diced mangos, diced avocados, cherry tomatoes, finely chopped red onion, and chopped fresh cilantro.
2. In a small bowl, whisk together lime juice, extra-virgin olive oil, salt, and black pepper to create the dressing. Add chopped jalapeño if desired for some heat.
3. Pour the dressing over the mango and avocado mixture.
4. Gently toss the salad until all ingredients are well coated with the dressing.
5. Taste and adjust seasoning if needed.
6. Refrigerate the salad for about 15-30 minutes before serving to enhance flavors.
7. Serve chilled as a refreshing side dish or enjoy it on its own.
8. Garnish with additional cilantro before serving if desired.

Roasted Beet and Goat Cheese Salad:

Ingredients:

- 3 medium-sized beets, peeled and diced
- 2 tablespoons olive oil
- Salt and black pepper to taste
- 4 cups mixed salad greens
- 1/2 cup goat cheese, crumbled
- 1/4 cup walnuts, toasted and chopped
- Balsamic glaze for drizzling (optional)

Instructions:

1. Preheat the oven to 400°F (200°C).
2. Toss diced beets with olive oil, salt, and black pepper in a bowl until well coated.
3. Spread the seasoned beets on a baking sheet in a single layer.
4. Roast the beets in the preheated oven for about 20-25 minutes or until they are tender and slightly caramelized. Stir halfway through the roasting time.
5. Allow the roasted beets to cool to room temperature.
6. In a large salad bowl, combine mixed salad greens, crumbled goat cheese, and toasted chopped walnuts.

7. Add the cooled roasted beets to the salad.

8. Drizzle with balsamic glaze if desired for an extra burst of flavor.

9. Toss the salad gently to combine all the ingredients.

10. Serve immediately as a side dish or a light, elegant appetizer.

Caprese Salad:

Ingredients:

- 4 large ripe tomatoes, sliced
- 1 pound fresh mozzarella cheese, sliced
- Fresh basil leaves
- Extra-virgin olive oil
- Balsamic glaze (optional)
- Salt and black pepper to taste

Instructions:

1. Arrange the tomato and mozzarella slices alternately on a serving platter.

2. Tuck fresh basil leaves between the tomato and mozzarella slices.

3. Drizzle extra-virgin olive oil over the salad.

4. If desired, add a touch of balsamic glaze for added sweetness and flavor.

5. Sprinkle salt and black pepper to taste.

6. Serve immediately to enjoy the freshness of the ingredients.

Broccoli and Almond Salad:

Ingredients:

- 4 cups broccoli florets, blanched
- 1/2 cup almonds, sliced and toasted
- 1/4 cup red onion, finely chopped
- 1/4 cup raisins or dried cranberries
- 1/4 cup feta cheese, crumbled
- 2 tablespoons olive oil

- 2 tablespoons red wine vinegar
- 1 tablespoon honey
- 1 teaspoon Dijon mustard
- Salt and black pepper to taste

Instructions:

1. Blanch the broccoli florets in boiling water for about 2-3 minutes, then transfer them to an ice bath to stop the cooking process. Drain and pat them dry.
2. In a large bowl, combine blanched broccoli, sliced and toasted almonds, finely chopped red onion, raisins or dried cranberries, and crumbled feta cheese.
3. In a small bowl, whisk together olive oil, red wine vinegar, honey, Dijon mustard, salt, and black pepper to create the dressing.
4. Pour the dressing over the broccoli mixture.
5. Toss the salad gently until all ingredients are well coated with the dressing.
6. Let the salad marinate for about 15-20 minutes in the refrigerator to allow the flavors to meld.
7. Serve chilled as a side dish or a light, nutritious meal.

Arugula and Fennel Salad:

Ingredients:

- 4 cups arugula, washed and dried
- 1 medium-sized fennel bulb, thinly sliced
- 1/2 cup cherry tomatoes, halved
- 1/4 cup shaved Parmesan cheese
- 2 tablespoons extra-virgin olive oil
- 1 tablespoon lemon juice
- 1 teaspoon Dijon mustard
- 1 teaspoon honey
- Salt and black pepper to taste

Instructions:

1. In a large salad bowl, combine arugula, thinly sliced fennel, cherry tomatoes, and shaved Parmesan cheese.
2. In a small bowl, whisk together extra-virgin olive oil, lemon juice, Dijon mustard, honey, salt, and black pepper to create the dressing.
3. Drizzle the dressing over the arugula and fennel mixture.
4. Toss the salad gently until all ingredients are well coated with the dressing.
5. Taste and adjust seasoning if needed.
6. Serve immediately as a refreshing side dish or a light, peppery salad.
7. Optionally, garnish with additional shaved Parmesan before serving.

Beverages;

Water with Lemon:

Ingredients:

- 1 glass of water
- 1 fresh lemon, sliced

Instructions:

1. Fill a glass with fresh, clean water.
2. Slice a lemon into thin rounds.
3. Squeeze a few lemon slices into the water for added flavor.
4. Drop the squeezed lemon slices into the water.
5. Stir gently or let the lemon infuse into the water naturally.
6. Optionally, add ice cubes for a refreshing chill.
7. Enjoy your revitalizing and hydrating Water with Lemon!

Green Tea:

Ingredients:

- 1 teaspoon green tea leaves or 1 green tea bag
- 1 cup hot water (not boiling, around 175°F or 80°C)

- Optional: Honey, lemon, or mint for flavor

Instructions:

1. Boil water and let it cool for a minute to reach the ideal temperature for green tea (around 175°F or 80°C).
2. Place the green tea leaves or tea bag into a teapot or a cup.
3. Pour the hot water over the tea leaves or tea bag.
4. Let the tea steep for 2-3 minutes. Steeping time may vary based on personal preference; longer steeping can result in a stronger flavor.
5. Remove the tea leaves or tea bag to prevent over-steeping and bitterness.
6. If desired, add honey, a slice of lemon, or a sprig of mint for additional flavor.
7. Stir gently, and enjoy your calming and antioxidant-rich cup of Green Tea!

Herbal Tea:

Ingredients:

- 1 tablespoon dried herbal tea blend or 1 herbal tea bag
- 1 cup hot water (boiling)
- Optional: Honey, fresh herbs, or citrus slices for flavor

Instructions:

1. Boil water and let it cool for a moment to around 212°F (100°C).
2. Place the dried herbal tea blend or herbal tea bag into a teapot or a cup.
3. Pour the hot water over the herbal tea.
4. Allow the herbal tea to steep for 5-7 minutes. Adjust steeping time based on personal preference for a stronger or milder flavor.
5. Remove the herbal tea blend or tea bag.
6. If desired, add honey for sweetness or enhance the flavor with fresh herbs like mint or citrus slices.
7. Stir gently and let the herbal tea cool for a minute before sipping.
8. Enjoy your soothing and aromatic cup of Herbal Tea!

Berry Smoothie:

Ingredients:

- 1 cup mixed berries (strawberries, blueberries, raspberries)
- 1 banana, peeled and sliced
- 1/2 cup Greek yogurt
- 1/2 cup almond milk (or any milk of your choice)
- 1 tablespoon honey or maple syrup (optional)
- Ice cubes (optional)

Instructions:

1. Place mixed berries, sliced banana, Greek yogurt, and almond milk in a blender.
2. If desired, add honey or maple syrup for sweetness.
3. Optional: Add ice cubes to make the smoothie colder and thicker.
4. Blend all the ingredients until smooth and creamy.
5. Taste the smoothie and adjust sweetness or thickness as needed by adding more honey, milk, or ice cubes.
6. Pour the berry smoothie into a glass.
7. Garnish with a few whole berries on top if desired.
8. Serve immediately and enjoy your delicious and nutritious Berry Smoothie!

Watermelon Cooler:

Ingredients:

- 4 cups seedless watermelon, diced
- 1 cup cold water
- Juice of 1 lime
- 2 tablespoons honey or agave syrup
- Ice cubes
- Fresh mint leaves for garnish

Instructions:

1. Place diced watermelon in a blender.
2. Add cold water, lime juice, and honey or agave syrup.
3. Blend the ingredients until smooth.

4. Strain the watermelon mixture through a fine mesh sieve or cheesecloth to remove any pulp. This step is optional if you prefer a pulpy texture.
5. Chill the watermelon juice in the refrigerator for at least 30 minutes.
6. Fill glasses with ice cubes.
7. Pour the chilled watermelon juice over the ice.
8. Garnish with fresh mint leaves.
9. Stir gently and serve your refreshing Watermelon Cooler immediately!

Cranberry Juice:

Ingredients:

- 2 cups fresh or frozen cranberries
- 4 cups water
- 1/2 to 3/4 cup granulated sugar (adjust to taste)
- Optional: Orange zest or a splash of orange juice for added flavor

Instructions:

1. Rinse the cranberries under cold water.
2. In a medium saucepan, combine cranberries and water.
3. Bring the mixture to a boil, then reduce the heat and let it simmer for about 10-15 minutes until the cranberries burst.
4. Mash the cranberries using a potato masher or the back of a spoon to release more flavor.
5. Strain the mixture through a fine mesh sieve or cheesecloth into a bowl to separate the liquid from the solids. You can use the back of a spoon to press out more juice.
6. Return the strained liquid to the saucepan.
7. Add sugar to the liquid and stir until completely dissolved. Adjust the sweetness to your liking.
8. Optional: Add orange zest or a splash of orange juice for extra flavor.
9. Let the cranberry juice cool to room temperature.
10. Transfer the cranberry juice to a pitcher and refrigerate until chilled.
11. Serve over ice and enjoy your homemade Cranberry Juice!

Fresh Vegetable Juice:

Ingredients:

- 3 medium-sized carrots, washed and trimmed
- 2 cucumbers, washed
- 3 stalks celery, washed
- 1 medium-sized beet, washed and peeled
- 1 large tomato, washed
- 1/2 bell pepper (red or yellow), washed and seeds removed
- Handful of spinach leaves, washed
- 1 small piece of ginger, peeled
- Optional: Lemon or lime for a citrusy kick
- Ice cubes (optional)

Instructions:

1. Wash and prepare all the vegetables and fruits.
2. Cut the carrots, cucumbers, celery, beet, tomato, bell pepper, and ginger into smaller pieces to fit into your juicer.
3. If your juicer has different settings, start with the softer vegetables and fruits, like spinach and cucumber.
4. Feed the vegetables and fruits through the juicer, collecting the extracted juice in a pitcher.
5. If using a blender, blend the vegetables with a bit of water and then strain the mixture to obtain the juice.
6. Optional: Squeeze in some fresh lemon or lime juice for added brightness.
7. Stir the juice well and refrigerate for a short time if you prefer it chilled.
8. If desired, serve over ice cubes for a refreshing touch.
9. Pour into glasses and enjoy your nutrient-packed Fresh Vegetable Juice!

Coconut Water:

Ingredients:

- 1 fresh coconut

Instructions:

1. Select a fresh coconut with no cracks or signs of mold. Shake it to ensure there is liquid inside.

2. Using a sturdy knife, carefully cut off the top of the coconut, creating a small opening. Be cautious when handling the knife.

3. Pour the coconut water into a clean glass or container. If the coconut water has bits of coconut meat, you can strain it using a fine mesh sieve or cheesecloth.

4. Optionally, use a coconut water extraction tool or a straw to sip directly from the coconut.

5. Chill the coconut water in the refrigerator if you prefer it cold.

6. Serve the fresh coconut water as a hydrating and refreshing beverage.

Iced Peppermint Tea:

Ingredients:

- 4 cups water
- 4-5 peppermint tea bags or a handful of fresh peppermint leaves
- 2-3 tablespoons honey or sweetener of your choice (optional)
- Ice cubes
- Fresh mint leaves for garnish (optional)
- Lemon slices for garnish (optional)

Instructions:

1. Boil 4 cups of water.

2. Place the peppermint tea bags or fresh peppermint leaves in a heatproof pitcher.

3. Pour the boiling water over the tea bags or leaves.

4. Allow the tea to steep for 5-7 minutes, or until it reaches your desired strength.

5. Remove the tea bags or strain out the peppermint leaves.

6. If desired, add honey or sweetener to the hot tea and stir until dissolved. Adjust sweetness to your liking.

7. Let the tea cool to room temperature, then refrigerate until chilled.

8. Fill glasses with ice cubes.

9. Pour the chilled peppermint tea over the ice.

10. Garnish with fresh mint leaves and lemon slices if desired.

11. Stir gently and serve your refreshing Iced Peppermint Tea.

Limeade:

Ingredients:
- 1 cup fresh lime juice (approximately 8-10 limes)
- 1 cup granulated sugar
- 4 cups cold water
- Ice cubes
- Lime slices for garnish (optional)
- Fresh mint leaves for garnish (optional)

Instructions:
1. Squeeze fresh limes to extract 1 cup of lime juice. This may require about 8-10 limes, depending on their size and juiciness.
2. In a pitcher, combine the fresh lime juice and granulated sugar.
3. Stir the mixture until the sugar dissolves, creating a lime syrup.
4. Add 4 cups of cold water to the lime syrup. Adjust the water quantity based on your preferred level of tartness.
5. Stir well to combine all the ingredients.
6. Taste the limeade and adjust the sweetness by adding more sugar if needed.
7. Refrigerate the limeade for at least 30 minutes to chill and allow the flavors to meld.
8. Fill glasses with ice cubes.
9. Pour the chilled limeade over the ice.
10. Garnish with lime slices and fresh mint leaves if desired.
11. Stir gently and serve your homemade Limeade for a refreshing and citrusy treat!

Cucumber Infused Water:

Ingredients:
- 1 medium cucumber, washed and thinly sliced
- 8 cups water
- Ice cubes (optional)
- Fresh mint leaves for garnish (optional)

Instructions:
1. Wash the cucumber thoroughly.

2. Slice the cucumber into thin rounds.

3. In a large pitcher, add the cucumber slices.

4. Pour 8 cups of water over the cucumber slices.

5. Optionally, add ice cubes for a chilled infusion.

6. Stir gently to distribute the cucumber slices evenly.

7. Refrigerate the infused water for at least 1-2 hours, allowing the flavors to meld.

8. Before serving, stir the cucumber water once more.

9. Pour the cucumber-infused water into glasses.

10. Garnish with fresh mint leaves if desired.

11. Serve and enjoy your refreshing Cucumber Infused Water!

Pineapple Ginger Smoothie:

Ingredients:
- 1 cup fresh or frozen pineapple chunks
- 1 banana, peeled and sliced
- 1/2 cup Greek yogurt
- 1/2 cup almond milk (or any milk of your choice)
- 1 tablespoon fresh ginger, peeled and grated
- 1 tablespoon honey or maple syrup (optional)
- Ice cubes (optional)

Instructions:
1. Place pineapple chunks, sliced banana, Greek yogurt, almond milk, grated ginger, and honey (if using) in a blender.
2. Add ice cubes if you want a colder and thicker smoothie.
3. Blend all the ingredients until smooth and creamy.
4. Taste the smoothie and adjust sweetness or thickness by adding more honey, milk, or ice cubes.
5. Pour the Pineapple Ginger Smoothie into a glass.
6. Garnish with a slice of pineapple or a sprinkle of grated ginger if desired.
7. Serve immediately and enjoy your tropical and invigorating smoothie!

CHAPTER 11: WEEKLY MEAL PLAN

Monday:

- **Breakfast: Scrambled eggs with spinach and tomatoes**

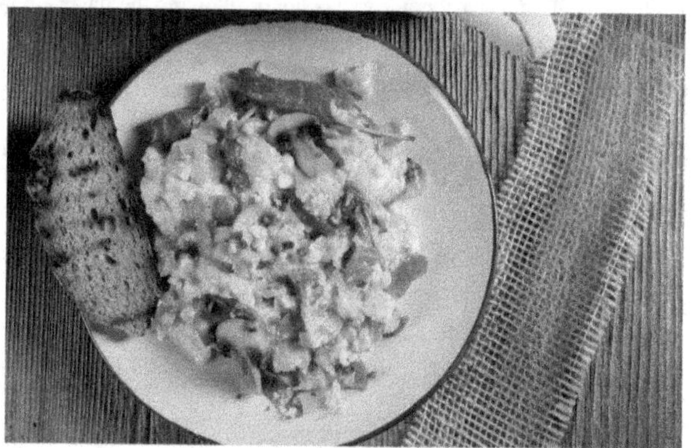

Ingredients:

- 4 eggs
- 1 cup fresh spinach, chopped
- 1 cup cherry tomatoes, halved
- 1/4 cup milk
- Salt and pepper to taste
- 2 tablespoons olive oil
- Optional: grated cheese for topping

Instructions:

- Heat olive oil in a skillet over medium heat.
- Add chopped spinach and halved cherry tomatoes to the skillet. Sauté until spinach wilts and tomatoes soften.
- In a bowl, whisk together eggs, milk, salt, and pepper until well combined.

- Pour the egg mixture over the spinach and tomatoes in the skillet.
- Gently stir the eggs, folding them over as they begin to set.
- Continue cooking and stirring until the eggs are fully cooked but still moist.
- If desired, sprinkle grated cheese over the scrambled eggs and cover the skillet until the cheese melts.
- Remove from heat and serve the scrambled eggs with spinach and tomatoes hot.
- Garnish with additional salt, pepper, or herbs to taste.
- **Snack: Apple slices with almond butter**

Ingredients:

- 2 apples, cored and sliced
- 1/4 cup almond butter
- Optional toppings: honey, cinnamon, or chopped nuts

Instructions:

- Wash and core the apples, then cut them into thin slices.
- Spread a generous layer of almond butter on each apple slice.
- If desired, drizzle honey over the almond butter or sprinkle with a pinch of cinnamon.
- For added crunch, top with chopped nuts such as almonds or walnuts.
- Arrange the apple slices on a serving plate or tray.
- **Lunch: Grilled chicken salad with mixed greens and olive oil dressing**

Ingredients:

For the Salad:

- 2 boneless, skinless chicken breasts
- 6 cups mixed salad greens (e.g., lettuce, arugula, spinach)
- 1 cup cherry tomatoes, halved
- 1 cucumber, sliced
- 1/2 red onion, thinly sliced
- 1/4 cup feta cheese, crumbled (optional)

For the Grilled Chicken Marinade:

- 2 tablespoons olive oil
- 2 cloves garlic, minced
- 1 teaspoon dried oregano
- Salt and pepper to taste

For the Olive Oil Dressing:

- 1/4 cup extra virgin olive oil
- 2 tablespoons balsamic vinegar
- 1 teaspoon Dijon mustard
- Salt and pepper to taste

Instructions:

- Marinate the Chicken:
    - In a bowl, mix olive oil, minced garlic, dried oregano, salt, and pepper.
    - Coat the chicken breasts with the marinade and let them marinate for at least 30 minutes.
- Grill the Chicken:
    - Preheat the grill or grill pan over medium-high heat.
    - Grill the marinated chicken breasts for about 6-8 minutes per side or until fully cooked.
    - Allow the chicken to rest for a few minutes before slicing it into thin strips.
- Prepare the Salad:
    - In a large bowl, combine the mixed greens, cherry tomatoes, cucumber, red onion, and feta cheese.
- Make the Olive Oil Dressing:
    - In a small bowl, whisk together extra virgin olive oil, balsamic vinegar, Dijon mustard, salt, and pepper.
- Assemble the Salad:
    - Arrange the grilled chicken strips on top of the mixed greens.
    - Drizzle the olive oil dressing over the salad.

- Serve:
    - Toss the salad gently to coat the ingredients with the dressing.
    - Serve the grilled chicken salad immediately, and enjoy a healthy and flavorful lunch!
- **Snack: Greek yogurt with berries**

Ingredients:

- 1 cup Greek yogurt (plain or flavored)
- 1/2 cup mixed berries (such as strawberries, blueberries, and raspberries)
- 1 tablespoon honey (optional)
- 2 tablespoons granola (optional)

Instructions:

- Prepare the Berries:
    - Wash the berries thoroughly and pat them dry with a paper towel.
- Assemble the Snack:
    - Spoon the Greek yogurt into a bowl or serving dish.
- Add the Berries:
    - Arrange the mixed berries on top of the Greek yogurt.
- Drizzle with Honey (Optional):
    - If you prefer a touch of sweetness, drizzle honey over the yogurt and berries.
- Optional Crunch with Granola:
    - For added texture, sprinkle granola over the yogurt and berries.
- Serve:
    - Enjoy this simple and refreshing Greek yogurt with berries snack immediately.
- **Dinner: Baked salmon with asparagus and quinoa**

Ingredients:

- 4 salmon fillets

- 1 bunch of asparagus, trimmed
- 1 cup quinoa
- 2 cups water or vegetable broth
- 2 tablespoons olive oil
- 2 cloves garlic, minced
- 1 lemon, sliced
- Salt and pepper to taste
- Fresh herbs (such as dill or parsley) for garnish

Instructions:

1. Preheat the oven to 400°F (200°C).
2. Rinse the quinoa under cold water. In a medium saucepan, combine the quinoa and water (or vegetable broth). Bring to a boil, then reduce heat, cover, and simmer for about 15 minutes or until the quinoa is cooked and water is absorbed. Fluff with a fork.
3. While the quinoa is cooking, arrange the salmon fillets and trimmed asparagus on a baking sheet lined with parchment paper. Drizzle olive oil over them and season with minced garlic, salt, and pepper. Place lemon slices on top.
4. Bake in the preheated oven for 15-20 minutes or until the salmon is cooked through and flakes easily with a fork. The asparagus should be tender yet crisp.
5. Serve the baked salmon and asparagus over a bed of quinoa. Garnish with fresh herbs and additional lemon slices if desired.

Tuesday:

- **Breakfast: Omelette with mushrooms, onions, and turkey**

Ingredients:

- 3 large eggs
- 1/2 cup mushrooms, sliced
- 1/4 cup onion, finely chopped

- 1/4 cup cooked turkey, diced
- Salt and pepper to taste
- 1 tablespoon olive oil or butter
- Optional: shredded cheese for topping

Instructions:

- In a bowl, beat the eggs and season with salt and pepper. Set aside.
- Heat olive oil or butter in a non-stick skillet over medium heat.
- Add the chopped onions and sliced mushrooms to the skillet. Sauté until the vegetables are tender and the mushrooms have released their moisture.
- Add the diced turkey to the skillet and cook until heated through.
- Push the vegetables and turkey to one side of the skillet, and pour the beaten eggs into the other side.
- Allow the eggs to set for a moment, then gently stir the vegetables and turkey into the eggs.
- Continue cooking, lifting the edges of the omelette to let the uncooked eggs flow underneath until the eggs are set but still moist.
- If desired, sprinkle shredded cheese over one half of the omelette.
- Fold the omelette in half, covering the filling. Cook for an additional minute to melt the cheese.
- Slide the omelette onto a plate and serve hot.
- **Snack: Handful of walnuts**

Ingredients:

- Walnuts

Instructions:

- Take a handful of walnuts, approximately one ounce (about 14 halves).
- Optionally, you can rinse the walnuts under cold water and pat them dry for a refreshing touch.
- Enjoy this simple and nutritious snack of walnuts.

- **Lunch: Stir-fried bok choy with lean beef and brown rice**

Ingredients:

- 1 lb lean beef, thinly sliced
- 4 cups bok choy, chopped
- 2 cups cooked brown rice
- 3 tablespoons soy sauce
- 1 tablespoon oyster sauce
- 1 tablespoon sesame oil
- 2 cloves garlic, minced
- 1 teaspoon fresh ginger, grated
- 2 tablespoons vegetable oil
- Salt and pepper to taste
- Optional: red pepper flakes for added spice
- Optional garnish: sliced green onions and sesame seeds

Instructions:

- In a bowl, marinate the thinly sliced beef with soy sauce, oyster sauce, minced garlic, and grated ginger. Allow it to marinate for at least 15 minutes.
- Heat vegetable oil in a large wok or skillet over medium-high heat.
- Add the marinated beef to the hot pan, stirring frequently until the beef is browned and cooked through. Remove the cooked beef from the pan and set aside.
- In the same pan, add a bit more oil if needed, and stir-fry the bok choy until it wilts but is still crisp, about 2-3 minutes.
- Return the cooked beef to the pan with the bok choy, and add sesame oil. Toss everything together until well combined. Season with salt, pepper, and optional red pepper flakes to taste.
- Serve the stir-fried beef and bok choy over a bed of cooked brown rice.
- Garnish with sliced green onions and sesame seeds if desired.

- **Snack: Orange slices**

Ingredients:

- 2 oranges

Instructions:

- Wash the oranges thoroughly.
- Slice off the top and bottom of each orange.
- Stand the orange on one of the flat ends and carefully cut away the peel and white pith, following the natural curve of the fruit.
- Once peeled, slice the oranges into rounds or wedges.
- Arrange the orange slices on a plate or in a bowl.
- Serve and enjoy this refreshing and naturally sweet snack.
- **Dinner: Shrimp and broccoli stir-fry with cauliflower rice**

Ingredients:

- 1 lb shrimp, peeled and deveined
- 3 cups broccoli florets
- 1 medium cauliflower, riced
- 3 tablespoons soy sauce
- 1 tablespoon oyster sauce
- 1 tablespoon sesame oil
- 2 tablespoons vegetable oil
- 2 cloves garlic, minced
- 1 teaspoon fresh ginger, grated
- Salt and pepper to taste
- Optional: red pepper flakes for added spice
- Optional garnish: sliced green onions and sesame seeds

Instructions:

1. In a bowl, combine shrimp with soy sauce, oyster sauce, minced garlic, and grated ginger. Allow it to marinate for about 15 minutes.

2. Heat vegetable oil in a large wok or skillet over medium-high heat.

3. Add the marinated shrimp to the hot pan, stirring frequently until the shrimp are pink and cooked through. Remove the cooked shrimp from the pan and set aside.

4. In the same pan, add a bit more oil if needed, and stir-fry the broccoli until it's crisp-tender, about 3-4 minutes.

5. Push the broccoli to the sides of the pan, add the riced cauliflower to the center, and stir-fry until the cauliflower is cooked but still has a slight crunch.

6. Return the cooked shrimp to the pan with the broccoli and cauliflower. Drizzle sesame oil over the mixture and toss everything together until well combined. Season with salt, pepper, and optional red pepper flakes to taste.

7. Serve the shrimp and broccoli stir-fry over a bed of cauliflower rice.

8. Garnish with sliced green onions and sesame seeds if desired.

Wednesday:

- **Breakfast: Smoothie with kale, banana, and flaxseed**

Ingredients:

- 1 cup kale leaves, stems removed
- 1 ripe banana
- 1 tablespoon ground flaxseed
- 1 cup almond milk (or any preferred milk)
- 1/2 cup Greek yogurt (optional for added creaminess)
- Ice cubes (optional)
- Honey or maple syrup for sweetness (optional)

Instructions:

- Wash the kale leaves thoroughly, and remove the stems.
- In a blender, combine the kale leaves, ripe banana, ground flaxseed, almond milk, and Greek yogurt (if using).

- Blend the ingredients until smooth and creamy. If the smoothie is too thick, you can add more almond milk to reach your desired consistency.
- Taste the smoothie and add honey or maple syrup if additional sweetness is desired.
- If you prefer a colder smoothie, add ice cubes to the blender and blend until smooth.
- Pour the kale, banana, and flaxseed smoothie into a glass.
- Optionally, garnish with a sprinkle of additional flaxseed on top.
- **Snack: Celery sticks with hummus**

Ingredients:

- Fresh celery stalks, washed and trimmed
- Hummus (store-bought or homemade)

Instructions:

- Cut the washed and trimmed celery stalks into manageable sticks, approximately 4-5 inches long.
- Spoon a generous amount of hummus into a small bowl or plate for dipping.
- Dip the celery sticks into the hummus, coating them with the creamy goodness.
- Enjoy this simple and healthy snack that combines the crispiness of celery with the rich flavor of hummus.
- **Lunch: Turkey lettuce wraps with avocado**

Ingredients:

- 1 lb ground turkey
- 1 tablespoon olive oil
- 1 teaspoon cumin
- 1 teaspoon chili powder
- 1/2 teaspoon garlic powder
- Salt and pepper to taste
- Iceberg or butter lettuce leaves, washed and separated

- 1 ripe avocado, sliced
- Salsa or diced tomatoes for topping
- Greek yogurt or sour cream for garnish (optional)
- Fresh cilantro leaves for garnish (optional)
- Lime wedges for serving

Instructions:

- In a skillet, heat olive oil over medium heat. Add ground turkey and cook until browned, breaking it apart with a spatula as it cooks.
- Season the turkey with cumin, chili powder, garlic powder, salt, and pepper. Stir well to evenly distribute the spices.
- Once the turkey is fully cooked and seasoned, remove the skillet from heat.
- Wash and separate the lettuce leaves to create cups for the wraps.
- Spoon the seasoned ground turkey into the lettuce cups.
- Top each lettuce wrap with slices of ripe avocado.
- Add a dollop of salsa or diced tomatoes on top.
- Optionally, garnish with Greek yogurt or sour cream and fresh cilantro leaves.
- Serve the turkey lettuce wraps with lime wedges on the side for a burst of citrus flavor.

- **Snack: Pineapple chunks**

Ingredients:

- Fresh pineapple, peeled and cored

Instructions:

- Start by selecting a ripe pineapple. Look for a pineapple with a sweet aroma and golden skin.
- Wash the pineapple under cold water.
- Cut off the top and bottom of the pineapple, creating stable ends.
- Stand the pineapple upright and carefully slice off the skin, removing any "eyes."
- Slice the peeled pineapple into chunks or bite-sized pieces.

- Place the pineapple chunks in a bowl or on a plate.
- Optionally, refrigerate the pineapple chunks for a refreshing and chilled snack.
- Enjoy the natural sweetness and juiciness of fresh pineapple as a delightful and healthy snack.
- **Dinner: Lamb chops with roasted sweet potatoes and green beans**

Ingredients:

- 4 lamb chops
- 3 medium sweet potatoes, peeled and diced
- 2 cups green beans, trimmed
- 3 tablespoons olive oil
- 3 cloves garlic, minced
- 1 teaspoon dried rosemary
- Salt and pepper to taste
- Optional: balsamic glaze for drizzling
- Fresh parsley for garnish

Instructions:

1. Preheat the oven to 400°F (200°C).
2. Place the diced sweet potatoes on a baking sheet. Drizzle with 2 tablespoons of olive oil, sprinkle minced garlic, dried rosemary, salt, and pepper. Toss to coat evenly.
3. Arrange the sweet potatoes in a single layer and roast in the preheated oven for about 20-25 minutes or until tender and slightly caramelized, turning once halfway through.
4. While the sweet potatoes are roasting, season the lamb chops with salt and pepper.
5. Heat the remaining 1 tablespoon of olive oil in a skillet over medium-high heat. Sear the lamb chops for about 3-4 minutes on each side or until browned and cooked to your desired doneness.

6. In the last 5 minutes of roasting the sweet potatoes, add the trimmed green beans to the baking sheet. Drizzle with a bit of olive oil and season with salt and pepper.

7. Once the lamb chops are cooked and the sweet potatoes and green beans are roasted, arrange them on a serving platter.

8. Optionally, drizzle with balsamic glaze for added flavor.

9. Garnish with fresh parsley

Thursday:

- **Breakfast: Quinoa porridge with berries**

Ingredients:

- 1/2 cup quinoa, rinsed
- 1 cup milk (dairy or plant-based)
- 1 cup water
- 2 tablespoons maple syrup or honey
- 1/2 teaspoon vanilla extract
- Pinch of salt
- Mixed berries (strawberries, blueberries, raspberries) for topping
- Nuts or seeds (such as almonds or chia seeds) for garnish

Instructions:

- Rinse the quinoa under cold water.
- In a saucepan, combine quinoa, milk, water, maple syrup (or honey), vanilla extract, and a pinch of salt.
- Bring the mixture to a boil, then reduce the heat to low, cover, and simmer for about 15 minutes or until the quinoa is cooked and the mixture thickens.
- Stir occasionally to prevent sticking and ensure even cooking.
- Once the quinoa porridge reaches your desired consistency, remove it from heat.
- Spoon the quinoa porridge into bowls.
- Top with mixed berries and garnish with nuts or seeds for added texture.

- Optionally, drizzle with additional maple syrup or honey for sweetness.
- **Snack: Cherry tomatoes with mozzarella cheese**

Ingredients:

- Cherry tomatoes
- Fresh mozzarella cheese, small balls or diced
- Fresh basil leaves
- Extra virgin olive oil
- Balsamic glaze (optional)
- Salt and pepper to taste

Instructions:

- Wash the cherry tomatoes and cut them in half.
- If using larger mozzarella balls, cut them into bite-sized pieces.
- On toothpicks or small skewers, thread a half cherry tomato, a piece of mozzarella, and a fresh basil leaf.
- Arrange the tomato, mozzarella, and basil skewers on a serving plate.
- Drizzle extra virgin olive oil over the skewers.
- Optionally, add a touch of balsamic glaze for extra flavor.
- Sprinkle salt and pepper to taste.
- Serve and enjoy this simple and refreshing snack that combines the sweetness of cherry tomatoes with the creamy goodness of mozzarella and the aromatic freshness of basil.
- **Lunch: Grilled tuna steak with mixed vegetables**

Ingredients:

- 2 tuna steaks
- 2 tablespoons soy sauce
- 1 tablespoon olive oil
- 1 tablespoon lemon juice
- 2 cloves garlic, minced

- 1 teaspoon Dijon mustard
- Salt and pepper to taste
- Mixed vegetables (bell peppers, zucchini, cherry tomatoes, etc.)
- 1 tablespoon balsamic vinegar
- Fresh herbs (such as thyme or rosemary) for garnish

Instructions:

- In a bowl, whisk together soy sauce, olive oil, lemon juice, minced garlic, Dijon mustard, salt, and pepper to create the marinade.
- Place the tuna steaks in a shallow dish and pour half of the marinade over them. Allow the tuna to marinate for at least 15 minutes.
- Preheat the grill to medium-high heat.
- In the meantime, prepare the mixed vegetables. Toss them in the remaining marinade, ensuring they are well coated.
- Thread the mixed vegetables onto skewers or use a grilling basket for easy cooking.
- Grill the tuna steaks for about 3-4 minutes per side or to your desired level of doneness.
- Grill the mixed vegetables until they are slightly charred and tender.
- Remove the tuna steaks and mixed vegetables from the grill.
- Drizzle the grilled vegetables with balsamic vinegar for extra flavor.
- Serve the grilled tuna steaks alongside the mixed vegetables.
- Garnish with fresh herbs.
- **Snack: Pear slices with almond slices**

Ingredients:

- Fresh pears, sliced
- Almond slices

Instructions:

- Wash and slice the pears into thin wedges or bite-sized pieces.

- Arrange the pear slices on a plate or serving dish.
- Sprinkle almond slices over the pear slices.
- Optionally, drizzle a small amount of honey over the pear and almond slices for added sweetness.
- Serve and enjoy this simple and nutritious snack that combines the natural sweetness of pears with the crunch of almond slices.
- **Dinner: Chicken and vegetable curry with basmati rice**

Ingredients:

- 1 lb boneless, skinless chicken thighs, cut into bite-sized pieces
- 2 tablespoons curry powder
- 1 teaspoon ground cumin
- 1 teaspoon ground coriander
- 1/2 teaspoon turmeric
- 1/2 teaspoon chili powder (adjust to taste)
- Salt and pepper to taste
- 2 tablespoons vegetable oil
- 1 onion, finely chopped
- 2 cloves garlic, minced
- 1 tablespoon fresh ginger, grated
- 1 can (14 oz) diced tomatoes
- 1 cup coconut milk
- 2 cups mixed vegetables (e.g., carrots, bell peppers, peas)
- Fresh cilantro for garnish
- Cooked basmati rice for serving

Instructions:

1. In a bowl, mix curry powder, ground cumin, ground coriander, turmeric, chili powder, salt, and pepper. Toss the chicken pieces in this spice mixture until well coated.

2. Heat vegetable oil in a large skillet or pot over medium-high heat.

3. Add chopped onions, minced garlic, and grated ginger to the hot oil. Sauté until the onions are soft and fragrant.

4. Add the spice-coated chicken to the skillet and brown on all sides.

5. Pour in the diced tomatoes with their juice, stirring to combine.

6. Add coconut milk to the mixture, bringing it to a simmer.

7. Stir in the mixed vegetables and continue simmering until the chicken is cooked through and the vegetables are tender.

8. Adjust seasoning if needed, and let the curry simmer for an additional 5-10 minutes to allow flavors to meld.

9. Serve the chicken and vegetable curry over cooked basmati rice.

10. Garnish with fresh cilantro.

Friday:

- **Breakfast: Greek yogurt parfait with granola and strawberries**

Ingredients:

- 1 cup Greek yogurt
- 1/2 cup granola
- 1 cup fresh strawberries, hulled and sliced
- Honey for drizzling (optional)

Instructions:

- In a glass or bowl, spoon a layer of Greek yogurt at the bottom.
- Add a layer of granola on top of the Greek yogurt.
- Place a layer of sliced strawberries over the granola.
- Repeat the layers until you reach the top of the glass or bowl.
- Optionally, drizzle honey over the top for added sweetness.
- Serve immediately and enjoy this delicious and nutritious Greek yogurt parfait with granola and strawberries for breakfast.

- **Snack: Mixed nuts (almonds, cashews, and walnuts)**

Ingredients:
- 1 cup mixed nuts (almonds, cashews, walnuts)
- 1/2 teaspoon olive oil
- 1/2 teaspoon sea salt
- Optional: pinch of cayenne pepper for a spicy kick

Instructions:
- Preheat the oven to 350°F (175°C).
- In a bowl, toss the mixed nuts with olive oil until they are evenly coated.
- Spread the nuts in a single layer on a baking sheet lined with parchment paper.
- Sprinkle sea salt (and optional cayenne pepper) over the nuts.
- Bake in the preheated oven for about 10-12 minutes, or until the nuts are lightly toasted, stirring once or twice during the baking time.
- Remove the nuts from the oven and let them cool completely before serving.
- Once cooled, transfer the mixed nuts to a bowl or store in an airtight container.
- Enjoy this simple and savory mixed nut snack that provides a satisfying crunch and a mix of healthy fats.
- **Lunch: Turkey and avocado salad with a lemon vinaigrette**

Ingredients:
- 2 cups cooked turkey, shredded or diced
- 2 avocados, peeled, pitted, and sliced
- 4 cups mixed salad greens (e.g., spinach, arugula, or mixed greens)
- 1 cup cherry tomatoes, halved
- 1/4 cup red onion, thinly sliced
- 1/4 cup feta cheese, crumbled (optional)
- 2 tablespoons fresh cilantro or parsley, chopped (optional)

For Lemon Vinaigrette:
- 3 tablespoons olive oil

- 1 tablespoon fresh lemon juice
- 1 teaspoon Dijon mustard
- 1 clove garlic, minced
- Salt and pepper to taste

Instructions:

- In a large salad bowl, combine the cooked turkey, sliced avocados, mixed salad greens, cherry tomatoes, red onion, and feta cheese (if using).
- In a small bowl or jar, whisk together the olive oil, fresh lemon juice, Dijon mustard, minced garlic, salt, and pepper to create the lemon vinaigrette.
- Drizzle the lemon vinaigrette over the salad ingredients.
- Toss the salad gently to ensure even coating of the dressing.
- Garnish with chopped cilantro or parsley if desired.
- Serve the turkey and avocado salad immediately.
- **Snack: Kiwi slices**

Ingredients:

- Fresh kiwi

Instructions:

- Wash and peel the kiwi.
- Slice the kiwi into thin rounds or bite-sized pieces.
- Optionally, you can also cut the slices into halves for smaller portions.
- Arrange the kiwi slices on a plate or in a bowl.
- Serve and enjoy this simple and nutritious snack with the natural sweetness of fresh kiwi.
- **Dinner: Baked cod with Brussels sprouts and wild rice**

Ingredients:

- 4 cod fillets
- 1 lb Brussels sprouts, trimmed and halved
- 1 cup wild rice, rinsed

- 2 1/2 cups vegetable or chicken broth
- 3 tablespoons olive oil
- 2 cloves garlic, minced
- 1 teaspoon dried thyme
- Salt and pepper to taste
- Lemon wedges for serving

Instructions:

1. Preheat the oven to 400°F (200°C).
2. In a baking dish, place the cod fillets. Drizzle with 1 tablespoon of olive oil and season with minced garlic, dried thyme, salt, and pepper.
3. In a separate baking dish, toss the halved Brussels sprouts with 2 tablespoons of olive oil, salt, and pepper.
4. Place both baking dishes in the preheated oven. Bake the cod for about 15-20 minutes or until it flakes easily with a fork. Roast the Brussels sprouts for about 20-25 minutes or until they are tender and lightly browned.
5. While the cod and Brussels sprouts are baking, rinse the wild rice under cold water.
6. In a saucepan, combine the rinsed wild rice and broth. Bring to a boil, then reduce the heat, cover, and simmer for about 40-45 minutes or until the rice is tender and the liquid is absorbed.
7. Fluff the cooked wild rice with a fork.
8. Serve the baked cod over a bed of wild rice with roasted Brussels sprouts on the side.
9. Garnish with lemon wedges for squeezing over the cod.

Saturday:

- **Breakfast: Frittata with spinach, feta cheese, and cherry tomatoes**

Ingredients:

- 6 large eggs
- 1 cup fresh spinach, chopped
- 1/2 cup feta cheese, crumbled
- 1 cup cherry tomatoes, halved
- 1/2 cup milk
- 1 tablespoon olive oil
- 1 small onion, finely chopped
- Salt and pepper to taste
- Fresh basil or parsley for garnish (optional)

Instructions:

- Preheat the oven to 375°F (190°C).
- In a bowl, whisk together eggs, milk, salt, and pepper.
- Heat olive oil in an oven-safe skillet over medium heat.
- Add chopped onion to the skillet and sauté until softened.
- Add chopped spinach to the skillet and cook until wilted.
- Pour the whisked egg mixture into the skillet, ensuring an even distribution of spinach and onion.
- Place halved cherry tomatoes evenly across the frittata.
- Sprinkle crumbled feta cheese over the top.
- Allow the edges of the frittata to set on the stove for a few minutes.
- Transfer the skillet to the preheated oven and bake for approximately 15-20 minutes or until the frittata is set and the top is lightly golden.
- Remove from the oven and let it cool for a few minutes.
- Optionally, garnish with fresh basil or parsley.
- Slice and serve your delicious spinach, feta, and cherry tomato frittata.
- **Snack: Carrot sticks with tzatziki**

Ingredients:

- Fresh carrots, washed and peeled

- Tzatziki sauce (store-bought or homemade)

Instructions:

- Cut the washed and peeled carrots into sticks or bite-sized pieces.
- Place the carrot sticks on a plate or in a snack container.
- Spoon tzatziki sauce into a small bowl for dipping.
- Dip the carrot sticks into the tzatziki sauce, ensuring they are well coated.
- Enjoy this crunchy and refreshing snack that combines the natural sweetness of carrots with the cool and tangy flavor of tzatziki.
- **Lunch: Quinoa salad with grilled chicken and assorted vegetables**

Ingredients:

- 1 cup quinoa, rinsed
- 2 cups water or vegetable broth
- 1 lb boneless, skinless chicken breasts
- 2 tablespoons olive oil
- Salt and pepper to taste
- 1 cup cherry tomatoes, halved
- 1 cucumber, diced
- 1 bell pepper (any color), diced
- 1/4 red onion, finely chopped
- 1/2 cup feta cheese, crumbled
- Fresh parsley or cilantro for garnish

For the Dressing:

- 3 tablespoons olive oil
- 2 tablespoons balsamic vinegar
- 1 teaspoon Dijon mustard
- Salt and pepper to taste

Instructions:

- In a saucepan, combine quinoa and water or vegetable broth. Bring to a boil, then reduce heat, cover, and simmer for about 15 minutes or until the quinoa is cooked and liquid is absorbed. Fluff with a fork and let it cool.
- Preheat the grill or grill pan over medium-high heat.
- Brush chicken breasts with olive oil and season with salt and pepper. Grill for about 6-8 minutes per side or until fully cooked.
- Let the grilled chicken rest for a few minutes, then slice it into strips.
- In a large bowl, combine cooked quinoa, grilled chicken strips, cherry tomatoes, cucumber, bell pepper, red onion, and feta cheese.
- In a small bowl, whisk together olive oil, balsamic vinegar, Dijon mustard, salt, and pepper to create the dressing.
- Pour the dressing over the quinoa salad and toss to coat evenly.
- Garnish with fresh parsley or cilantro.
- Serve this vibrant and nutritious quinoa salad with grilled chicken and assorted vegetables for a delicious and satisfying lunch.
- **Snack: Mango slices**

Ingredients:
- Ripe mango

Instructions:
- Wash the mango under cold water.
- Cut off both ends of the mango, creating stable flat surfaces.
- Stand the mango upright on one of the flat ends.
- With a sharp knife, carefully peel the skin off the mango, following the contour of the fruit.
- Once peeled, slice the mango into thin or thick slices, depending on your preference.
- Arrange the mango slices on a plate or in a bowl.

- Optionally, sprinkle a pinch of chili powder or a squeeze of lime juice for added flavor.
- Serve and enjoy this refreshing and naturally sweet snack.
- **Dinner: Stir-fried shrimp with broccoli and brown rice**

Ingredients:

- 1 lb large shrimp, peeled and deveined
- 2 cups broccoli florets
- 1 cup brown rice, cooked
- 3 tablespoons soy sauce
- 1 tablespoon oyster sauce
- 1 tablespoon sesame oil
- 2 tablespoons vegetable oil
- 2 cloves garlic, minced
- 1 teaspoon fresh ginger, grated
- Salt and pepper to taste
- Optional: red pepper flakes for added spice
- Optional garnish: sliced green onions and sesame seeds

Instructions:

1. In a bowl, mix the shrimp with soy sauce, oyster sauce, minced garlic, and grated ginger. Allow it to marinate for about 15 minutes.
2. Heat vegetable oil in a wok or large skillet over medium-high heat.
3. Add the marinated shrimp to the hot pan, stirring frequently until the shrimp turn pink and are cooked through. Remove the cooked shrimp from the pan and set aside.
4. In the same pan, add a bit more oil if needed, and stir-fry the broccoli until it's crisp-tender.
5. Return the cooked shrimp to the pan with the broccoli.

6. Drizzle sesame oil over the shrimp and broccoli mixture. Toss everything together until well combined.

7. Season with salt, pepper, and optional red pepper flakes to taste.

8. Serve the stir-fried shrimp and broccoli over a bed of cooked brown rice.

9. Garnish with sliced green onions and sesame seeds if desired.

Sunday:

- **Breakfast: Whole grain toast with avocado and poached eggs**

Ingredients:

- 2 slices of whole grain bread, toasted
- 1 ripe avocado
- 2 large eggs
- Salt and pepper to taste
- Optional toppings: red pepper flakes, paprika, or chopped herbs (e.g., chives or parsley)

Instructions:

- Toast the whole grain bread slices to your desired level of crispiness.
- While the bread is toasting, cut the ripe avocado in half, remove the pit, and scoop the flesh into a bowl. Mash the avocado with a fork and season with salt and pepper to taste.
- Poach the eggs: Bring a small pot of water to a gentle simmer. Crack each egg into a separate bowl. Create a gentle whirlpool in the simmering water and carefully slide one egg into the center. Poach each egg for about 3-4 minutes until the whites are set but the yolks are still runny. Remove with a slotted spoon and drain excess water.
- Spread the mashed avocado evenly over the toasted whole grain bread slices.
- Place a poached egg on top of each avocado-covered toast.
- Season the poached eggs with a sprinkle of salt and pepper.

- Optionally, add toppings like red pepper flakes, paprika, or chopped herbs for extra flavor.
- Serve the whole grain toast with avocado and poached eggs immediately.
- **Snack: Cottage cheese with pineapple chunks**

Ingredients:

- Cottage cheese
- Fresh pineapple, peeled and diced

Instructions:

- In a bowl, scoop desired portions of cottage cheese.
- Wash and peel the pineapple, then dice it into bite-sized chunks.
- Add the pineapple chunks to the bowl of cottage cheese.
- Gently mix the cottage cheese and pineapple until well combined.
- Optionally, refrigerate for a short time to chill before serving.
- Enjoy this quick and nutritious snack of cottage cheese with sweet and tangy pineapple chunks.
- **Lunch: Beef and vegetable kebabs with quinoa**

Ingredients:

- 1 lb beef sirloin or tenderloin, cut into cubes
- 1 bell pepper, cut into chunks
- 1 zucchini, sliced
- 1 red onion, cut into wedges
- Cherry tomatoes
- 1 cup quinoa, rinsed
- 2 cups water or beef broth
- 3 tablespoons olive oil
- 2 cloves garlic, minced
- 1 teaspoon dried oregano
- Salt and pepper to taste

- Wooden or metal skewers

Instructions:

- In a bowl, combine beef cubes with olive oil, minced garlic, dried oregano, salt, and pepper. Allow it to marinate for at least 15 minutes.
- Preheat the grill or grill pan to medium-high heat.
- Thread marinated beef cubes, bell pepper chunks, zucchini slices, red onion wedges, and cherry tomatoes onto skewers, alternating the ingredients.
- Grill the kebabs for about 10-15 minutes, turning occasionally, or until the beef is cooked to your liking and the vegetables are tender and slightly charred.
- While the kebabs are grilling, rinse quinoa under cold water.
- In a saucepan, combine quinoa with water or beef broth. Bring to a boil, then reduce heat, cover, and simmer for about 15-20 minutes or until the quinoa is cooked and liquid is absorbed. Fluff with a fork.
- Serve the beef and vegetable kebabs over a bed of cooked quinoa.
- **Snack: Blueberries**

Ingredients:

- Fresh blueberries

Instructions:

- Wash the blueberries under cold water.
- Drain any excess water using a colander or paper towel.
- Place the blueberries in a bowl or serve them directly in a snack container.
- Enjoy this simple and nutritious snack of fresh blueberries.
- **Dinner: Grilled halibut with roasted sweet potato wedges and green beans**

Ingredients:

- 4 halibut fillets
- 4 cups sweet potatoes, peeled and cut into wedges
- 2 cups green beans, trimmed

- 3 tablespoons olive oil
- 1 teaspoon smoked paprika
- 1 teaspoon garlic powder
- Salt and pepper to taste
- Lemon wedges for serving
- Fresh parsley for garnish

Instructions:

1. Preheat the grill to medium-high heat.
2. In a bowl, toss sweet potato wedges with 2 tablespoons of olive oil, smoked paprika, garlic powder, salt, and pepper until well coated.
3. Place the sweet potato wedges on a baking sheet or in a grill-safe pan.
4. Grill the sweet potato wedges for about 15-20 minutes or until they are tender and lightly browned, turning occasionally.
5. In a separate bowl, toss green beans with 1 tablespoon of olive oil, salt, and pepper.
6. Grill the halibut fillets for about 4-5 minutes per side or until the fish is cooked through and flakes easily with a fork.
7. In the last 5 minutes of grilling, add the seasoned green beans to the grill. Grill until they are crisp-tender.
8. Arrange grilled halibut, sweet potato wedges, and green beans on a serving platter.
9. Garnish with fresh parsley and serve with lemon wedges on the side.

GROCERY SHOPPING TIPS

1. Plan ahead by outlining your weekly meals and creating a shopping list. This reduces impulse purchases and ensures you have all of the necessities.
2. To find fresh veggies, lean meats, and dairy, shop the outer aisles of the supermarket store. This allows you to avoid processed and unhealthy products.
3. Choose a variety of colorful fruits and veggies. Fresh, in-season produce contains more nutrients and flavors.

4. Prioritize lean proteins such as poultry, fish, and lamb. When grass-fed or organic options are available, consider them.

5. Include omega-3-rich fish like salmon and mackerel in your diet. For the best nutritional value, use wild-caught kinds.

6. Read food labels to ensure they are compatible with the Blood Type O Diet. Avoid products containing additives, artificial colors, and unneeded preservatives.

7. Choose blood type-friendly herbs and spices, such as ginger, turmeric, and parsley, to enhance flavor without sacrificing health.

8. When shopping for grains, choose whole grains such as brown rice and quinoa. Look for alternatives that match your blood type.

9. Add nuts and seeds to your shopping for a nutritious snack. Almonds, walnuts, and flaxseeds are great options.

10. When incorporating dairy into your diet, go for goat or sheep milk products. Consider alternatives such as almond or coconut milk.

11. Avoid too processed and packaged foods. A Blood Type O Diet is based on fresh, natural foods.

12. Shop Seasonally: Make use of seasonal produce. It is generally less expensive and more nutritious.

13. Stay hydrated by consuming water-rich fruits and vegetables and drinking plenty of water.

14. Be flexible in your plan. If a specific item isn't available, consider alternatives that still meet your dietary criteria.

EATING OUT ON THE BLOOD TYPE O DIET

1. Plan ahead of time by researching restaurant menus online. This enables you to find Blood Type O-friendly options and make informed decisions.

2. Prioritize Protein: Choose lean options such as grilled chicken, turkey, fish, or lamb. These are consistent with the Blood Type O Diet.

3. Embrace veggies: Choose vegetable-rich recipes with leafy greens, broccoli, and other healthy veggies.

4. Customize Your Order: Ask for adjustments. Many restaurants are willing to accommodate dietary restrictions, such as switching sides or changing cooking methods.

5. To adhere to the Blood Type O Diet, avoid using sauces and dressings that may include incompatible substances. Ask for them on the side to keep your intake under control.

6. Grain Consciousness: Make sensible choices when eating grains. Choose whole grains such as brown rice or quinoa over ones that are less suitable with your blood type.

7. For nutritious snacks while waiting for your main course, try nuts, olives, or a small salad.

8. Maintain proper hydration by drinking water, herbal teas, or sugar-free beverages. This keeps you hydrated without affecting your diet.

9. Portion Control: Be mindful of portion sizes. To keep your food intake under control, consider sharing dishes or carrying leftovers.

10. Communicate Your Dietary Needs: If in doubt, inform the personnel about your dietary restrictions. Many eateries are willing to accept customised orders.

11. Practice mindfulness by eating slowly and savoring each bite. This not only improves your dining experience, but it also allows you to recognise when you're satisfied.

12. To satisfy your sweet taste, choose fruit-based or low-sugar treats. Consider sharing a taste to avoid overindulgence.

COOKING TIPS AND TECHNIQUES

1. Consider grilling or roasting lean foods such as chicken, turkey, fish, and lamb. This improves flavors without adding fat.

2. Use olive or flaxseed oil to stir-fry veggies, lean meats, and shellfish for added health benefits. This approach preserves nutrition while adding a wonderful crispness.

3. Marinate proteins using blood type-friendly herbs, spices, and acidic seasonings. This not only adds flavor but also aids in tenderization.

4. Steaming veggies helps preserve their nutrients. It's an easy and healthful technique to supplement the Blood Type O Diet.

5. Experiment With Blood Type-Friendly Herbs:

6. Explore herbs like ginger, turmeric, and parsley to enhance the flavour and health benefits of your recipes.

7. Smart Grain Swap: Use brown rice or quinoa instead. Experiment with options that are appropriate for the Blood Type O profile.

8. Create Nutrient-Dense Smoothies: Incorporate blood type-friendly fruits and vegetables for a simple and nutritious meal.

9. Prioritize fresh, seasonal produce. It not only improves flavors, but it also helps the Blood Type O Diet achieve its nutritional goals.

10. To save time on meal preparation, batch cook lean proteins, veggies, and grains.

11. Season with low-sodium soy sauce, miso, and other blood type-friendly ingredients to improve flavor without compromising health.

12. Cauliflower is a flexible alternative for grains and potatoes. It's a low-carb option that works well with the Blood Type O Diet.

13. Make your own dressings with blood type-friendly oils, herbs, and vinegars to enhance salads without adding unnecessary ingredients.

14. For Blood Type O persons, a balanced meal with lean protein, veggies, and healthy fats is recommended to suit their nutritional needs.

15. Diverse ethnic cuisines, such as Mediterranean or Asian, can complement the Blood Type O Diet and add variety to meals.

9 798877 743519